MULTISKILLING:

Electrocardiography

FOR THE HEALTH CARE PROVIDER

DEDICATION

For my late father, Carlos T. Brisendine, who is always in my thoughts.

ACKNOWLEDGMENTS

Continuing thanks and deepest appreciation to my companion, R. Miller; my parents, Stan and Anna Folda; my sisters, Terri Brisendine and Karla Popp; my dearest encouraging friends, Tracy Hedges and Linda Coleman; and my children, Brian Wasner, Jennifer Littler, and Melissa Compton, for their love and continual support.

Appreciation is expressed to the following practitioners and educators for their critical reviews of the manuscript:

Vicki Barclay, West Kentucky Technical College, Paducah, KY

Jennifer L. Barr, Sinclair Community College, Dayton, OH

Kenneth M. Bretl, College of DuPage, Glen Ellyn, IL

Beverly M. Kovanda, PhD, Columbus State Community College, Columbus, OH

Dawn Madl, Northeast Wisconsin Technical College, Green Bay, WI

MULTISKILLING:

Electrocardiography

FOR THE HEALTH CARE PROVIDER

Karen J. Brisendine, BS, MS, RVT
Mt. Carmel Medical Center, Columbus, OH

Beverly M. Kovanda
PhD, MS, MT (ASCP), CLP (NCA)
Series Editor

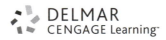

DELMAR
CENGAGE Learning™

Australia • Brazil • Japan • Korea • Mexico • Singapore • Spain • United Kingdom • United States

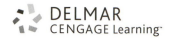

**Multiskilling: Electrocardiography
for the Health Care Provider**
Karen J. Brisendine

Publisher: Susan Simpfenderfer

Acquisitions Editor: Dawn Gerrain

Developmental Editor: Marjorie A. Bruce

Project Editor: Brooke Graves/Graves Editorial
    Service

Team Assistant: Sandra Bruce

Art and Design Coordinator: Vincent S. Berger

Production Coordinator: John Mickelbank

Marketing Manager: Katherine Slezak

Marketing Coordinator: Glenna Stanfield

Editorial Assistant: Donna L. Leto

For product information and technology assistance, contact us at
Cengage Learning Customer & Sales Support, 1-800-354-9706

For permission to use material from this text or product,
submit all requests online at **www.cengage.com/permissions**
Further permissions questions can be emailed to
permissionrequest@cengage.com

Library of Congress Control Number: 9737683

ISBN-13: 978-0-8273-8522-1

ISBN-10: 0-8273-8522-6

Delmar
Executive Woods
5 Maxwell Drive
Clifton Park, NY 12065-2919
USA

Cengage Learning is a leading provider of customized learning solutions with
office locations around the globe, including Singapore, the United Kingdom,
Australia, Mexico, Brazil, and Japan. Locate your local office at
www.cengage.com/global

Cengage Learning products are represented in Canada by Nelson Education, Ltd.

To learn more about Delmar, visit **www.cengage.com/delmar**

Purchase any of our products at your local bookstore or at our preferred online
store **www.cengagebrain.com**

Notice to the Reader

Publisher does not warrant or guarantee any of the products described herein or perform any independent
analysis in connection with any of the product information contained herein. Publisher does not assume,
and expressly disclaims, any obligation to obtain and include information other than that provided to it by
the manufacturer. The reader is expressly warned to consider and adopt all safety precautions that might be
indicated by the activities described herein and to avoid all potential hazards. By following the instructions
contained herein, the reader willingly assumes all risks in connection with such instructions. The publisher
makes no representations or warranties of any kind, including but not limited to, the warranties of fitness for
particular purpose or merchantability, nor are any such representations implied with respect to the material set
forth herein, and the publisher takes no responsibility with respect to such material. The publisher shall not be
liable for any special, consequential, or exemplary damages resulting, in whole or part, from the readers' use of,
or reliance upon, this material.

Printed in the United States of America
17 18 19 20 21 22 14 13 12 11 10

MESSAGE FROM THE SERIES EDITOR

The Multiskilling for Health Care Providers series consists of the *Patient Care: Basic Skills for the Health Care Provider* core text and many separate modular texts. The Multiskilling series offers a comprehensive vision of the diversity and many implications of multiskilling, whether in an acute care setting, home care, hospice, ambulatory setting, long-term care facility, or physician's office. The core text and module subjects have been identified through research as key topics in multiskilling and patient care training across the nation.

The framework for this series is found in the historic evolution of multiskilling, the National Health Care Skill Standards, and 13 years of personal experience in developing academic material and successfully training thousands of multiskilled health care providers in a multitude of nursing and allied health skill areas. The concept referred to as *multiskilling, crosstraining,* and (more recently) *patient care skills* began to gain national awareness in the mid-1980s, as pressures for cost containment in health care intensified. Institutions began to focus on more efficient use of personnel for economic survival. The implications of managed care are far-reaching.

In 1994, the National Health Care Skill Standards were developed through a national collaborative effort of health care organizations, professional organizations, schools, and colleges of higher education. By implementing these standards, we can more effectively serve the needs of a diverse client population and maintain quality care, while increasing the efficiency of staff utilization. Health care costs can be contained; the new technology, which is changing how and where health care is delivered, can be prudently applied. We believe that the skill standards are important and so their intent has been incorporated into the entire series.

The core text, *Patient Care: Basic Skills for the Health Care Provider,* meets the OBRA requirements for basic patient care skills. These skills are required of every health care provider who undertakes client care, regardless of the institutional setting or professional affiliation.

We believe that the core-text-plus-modules concept is the only rational approach to meeting the vastly different academic and training needs in multiskilling, as we re-engineer careers in all health care settings. The modules are flexible, well written, and academically sound. The modular approach is cost-effective. A health care worker's skills can be developed based upon individual goals, institutional needs for retraining, or specific career development. Colleges, hospitals, other health care agencies, technical and career schools, and "tech prep" programs need only purchase the modules that address their unique, customized academic and training needs. Because multiskilling is market-driven, other modules continue to be developed as health care needs are identified and evolve.

The modules are written by credentialed experts in each content area and multiskilling education. They have identified essential and appropriate nursing and allied health skills that can be accurately and safely performed by nonprofessionals to enhance the quality of patient care.

The depth of theory and skills in each module goes beyond other texts, which are usually written from the perspective of one profession rather than by specialists in each identifiable allied health and nursing area. We believe that this principle provides a stronger basis for instruction and facilitates a higher level of quality patient care.

The material in each module is organized in a clear, concise, straightforward manner to make learning easier, because health care institutions are demanding shorter—but intensified—training periods. The pedagogical features enhance retention and simplify learning.

We believe that the Multiskilling series combines the knowledge, experience, successes, and expertise of all of the authors. It provides the tools and flexibility to custom-design a curriculum that truly meets worker/student professional goals, augments valuable skills, and strengthens employability, not only now but as we prepare for the 21st century.

Beverly M. Kovanda, Ph.D., M.S., M.T. (ASCP), C.L.P. (NCA)
Coordinator/Professor
Multicompetency Health Technology

DELMAR'S MULTISKILLING SERIES

Patient Care: Basic Skills for the Health Care Provider
Multiskilling: Advanced Patient Care Skills for the Health Care Provider
Multiskilling: Phlebotomy Collection Procedures for the Health Care Provider
Multiskilling: Electrocardiography for the Health Care Provider
Multiskilling: Respiratory Care for the Health Care Provider
Multiskilling: Point of Care Testing-Capillary Puncture for the Health Care Provider

Modules Coming Soon:

Multiskilling: Waived Lab Testing for the Health Care Provider
Multiskilling: Team Building for the Health Care Provider
Multiskilling: Health Unit Coordinator for the Health Care Provider
Multiskilling: Physical Therapy/Rehabilitation Aide for the Health Care Provider
Multiskilling: Dietetic Aide for the Health Care Provider
Multiskilling: Basic Life Support for the Health Care Provider

Table of CONTENTS

EVOLVING ROLE OF HEALTH CARE AND THE ELECTROCARDIOGRAPHER

Health care has acquired a national focus and is undergoing rapid change. Case management has evolved as the new strategy or method for providing health care that is both efficient and of superior clinical quality. It is multidisciplinary care that focuses on patient outcomes and communication among members of the health care team.

Transformation of the health care industry affects every facet of the world. The search for the best quality care at optimal cost has established best care protocols and a simplification of numerous procedures. Creation of the new health care delivery system has resulted in dramatically improved client satisfaction ratings, increased client-family information and involvement in the plan of care, and decreased lengths of stay in inpatient settings. The client becomes the focus for the existence of health care. Multiskilling prevents confusion, a lack of continuity, and impersonal care; eliminates idle time of staff; and improves turnaround (response) time for procedures.

SKILLS NEEDED BY THE MULTISKILLED HEALTH CARE PROVIDER

Multiskilling of health care providers is essential for a future care delivery system that provides superior clinical quality and cost-effective outcomes. Although the ECG is an invaluable test, the diagnostic quality depends on the health care provider performing the ECG.

Multiskilling demands totally empowered, self-directed individuals. The patient-focused care concept requires self-governance and a broadening of authority and responsibility to perform as a productive health care team member. Essential qualities include:

- Excellent communication skills
- Group skills and cooperation
- Ability to resolve conflicts
- Adaptability to any situation and environment
- Continuous improvement

This module helps prepare health care providers to perform diagnostic ECGs by discussing anatomy, physiology of circulation, conduction principles, the cardiac cycle and the normal ECG complex, skin preparation and proper lead placement, artifact, required information and documentation on the ECG, and operation of equipment, maintenance, and trouble shooting. After reading this text, the health care provider will possess a basic understanding of ECG interpretation concerning dysrhythmia recognition, while performing the highest quality, diagnostic ECG possible to effectively evaluate cardiac status.

HISTORY OF THE ECG

The ECG is a diagnostic procedure that records electrical signals from the heart onto a paper strip. The pattern of these signals can tell a physician whether the heart is normal, experiencing electrical problems, under strain, or damaged. Before invention of the ECG, heart action could be observed only by direct contact with the open, exposed chest. The invention of the electrode by Augustus Waller in 1887 allowed electrical currents to be measured through intact skin.

Then, in 1903, Willem Einthoven was awarded the Nobel Prize for his invention of the electrocardiograph machine. The electrocardiogram, abbreviated ECG or EKG from the German *electrokardiogram,* is the graphic representation of electrical activity. Einthoven used a simple galvanometer–quartz string combination to sense or detect the electrical activating wave of the heart from electrodes placed on the surface of the body.

The first ECG machine consisted of a fine quartz wire suspended in a magnetic field. The wire was deflected either positively or negatively when subjected to an electrical current. The ECG recorded the passage of the electric wave across the chambers of the heart and through various nerve branches and measured progress of the wave through the heart with great accuracy. Einthoven developed criteria for the normal ECG; named the waves P, QRS, and T; and established the positions for electrode placement on the body.

IMPORTANCE AND USE OF ECG IN VARIOUS SETTINGS

According to Thaler (1995):

> The EKG is a tool of remarkable clinical power, remarkable for both the ease with which it can be mastered and for the extraordinary range of situations in which it can provide helpful and, frequently, even critical information. One glance at an EKG can diagnose an evolving myocardial infarction, identify a potentially life-threatening arrhythmia, pinpoint the chronic effects of sustained hypertension or the acute effects of a massive pulmonary embolism, or simply provide a measure of reassurance to someone who wants to begin an exercise program.

ECG is the most frequently utilized procedure for the diagnosis of heart disease. Electrocardiography is a unique technology providing essential and valuable knowledge not easily acquired by other methods. The ECG is safe, with no risk to the patient; it is uncomplicated and reproducible for serial examinations at relatively minimal cost.

A publication by the American College of Cardiologists (Fisch, 1995) stated:

> The electrocardiogram (ECG) has the following utilities: It may serve as an independent marker of myocardial disease; it may reflect anatomic, electrophysiologic, metabolic and hemodynamic alterations; it provides information that is essential for the proper diagnosis of and therapy for a variety of cardiac disorders; and it is without equal as a method for the diagnosis of arrhythmias.

CHAPTER 1

Basic Principles of the Cardiovascular System

OVERVIEW

A functional cardiovascular system is vital to life. Without blood circulation, the body cells would lack oxygen and nutrient supplies. Accumulated metabolic wastes would result in cell death. The heart performs as a pump and is responsible for the circulation of blood through the blood vessels. Heart contraction is a mechanical event triggered by electrical activation. This electrical activity of the heart may be transmitted externally through the skin during the cardiac cycle of systole and diastole. The ECG is a graphic representation of the electrical activity of the heart.

ANATOMY OF THE HEART

Location

The heart is a four-chambered pump located between the lungs in the middle of the chest. This remarkable, muscular organ weighs less than a pound and is approximately the size of a closed fist. Anatomically, the heart is located within the **mediastinum** and is bordered anteriorly by the **sternum,** posteriorly by the spine, and laterally by the lungs. The base of the heart attaches to several large blood vessels and lies beneath the second rib; the distal end extends downward to the left and terminates as a bluntly pointed **apex** at the fifth **intercostal space** (Figure 1-1).

Chambers

The valves and the **septum** separate the four chambers of the heart into the right and left **atria** and **ventricles** (Figure 1-2). The relatively thin-walled upper atria function as collecting and loading chambers, holding blood being returned to the heart. The thick-walled lower ventricles are the larger pumping chambers, expelling blood from the heart with each contraction. Pumping freshly oxygenated blood into the aorta and then throughout the body, the left side of the heart performs harder. Although pumping the same quantity of blood as the left heart, the right heart remains thinner because the blood is sent only a short distance—to the lungs for oxygenation.

- **mediastinum:** region of the thoracic cavity containing the heart and blood vessels, lying between the sternum and vertebral column and separating the lungs
- **sternum:** the breastbone
- **apex:** distal tip of the heart, located between the fifth and sixth ribs just below the left nipple
- **intercostal space:** the space between the ribs
- **septum:** a dividing wall between the atria or between the ventricles of the heart
- **atria (plural); atrium (singular):** upper, collecting chambers of the heart
- **ventricles:** lower, pumping chambers of the heart

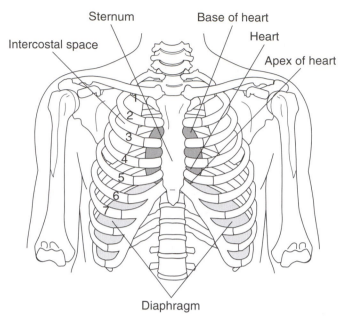

Sternum

Base of heart

Intercostal space

Heart

Apex of heart

1

2

3

4

5

6

Diaphragm

Figure 1-1   Heart location in the body

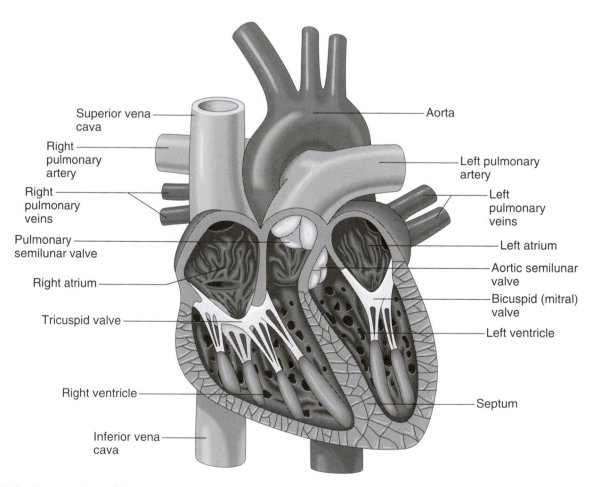

Superior vena cava

Aorta

Right pulmonary artery

Left pulmonary artery

Right pulmonary veins

Left pulmonary veins

Pulmonary semilunar valve

Left atrium

Right atrium

Aortic semilunar valve

Tricuspid valve

Bicuspid (mitral) valve

Left ventricle

Right ventricle

Septum

Inferior vena cava

Figure 1-2   Cross-section of the heart

■ **tricuspid valve:** *three-leaflet heart valve, located between the right atrium and ventricle*

■ **mitral valve:** *two-leaflet cardiac valve, situated between the left atrium and ventricle; also known as the bicuspid valve*

■ **pulmonary semilunar valve:** *heart valve positioned between the right ventricle and pulmonary artery*

■ **aortic valve:** *cardiac valve controlling flow between the left ventricle and aorta*

■ **chordae tendineae:** *strong, fibrous strings attached to cardiac valves and papillary muscles*

■ **endocardium:** *inner layer of cardiac muscle cells*

Valves

Strategically placed valves prevent the backflow of blood between the atria and ventricles. Cardiac valves control the direction of blood flow through the heart. The **tricuspid valve,** located between the right atrium and right ventricle, and the **mitral valve,** located between the left atrium and left ventricle, control the inflow of blood into the heart. The **pulmonary semilunar valve** monitors the outflow of blood between the right ventricle and the pulmonary artery; the **aortic valve** connects the outflow tract of the left ventricle with the aorta. The opening and closing of the valves produces the sound of the heartbeat heard with the stethoscope. Strong, fibrous, string-like tissues, the **chordae tendineae,** originate from small mounds of muscle tissue and permit opening and closing of the valves.

Cardiac Wall Layers

The **endocardium, myocardium,** and **epicardium** are the three layers of the heart muscle (Figure 1-3).

Endocardium

The endocardium is a layer of smooth cells lining the inner surface and cavities of the heart and the valves. Endocardium consists of a membrane composed of connective tissue and highly specialized cardiac muscle fibers called **Purkinje fibers.**

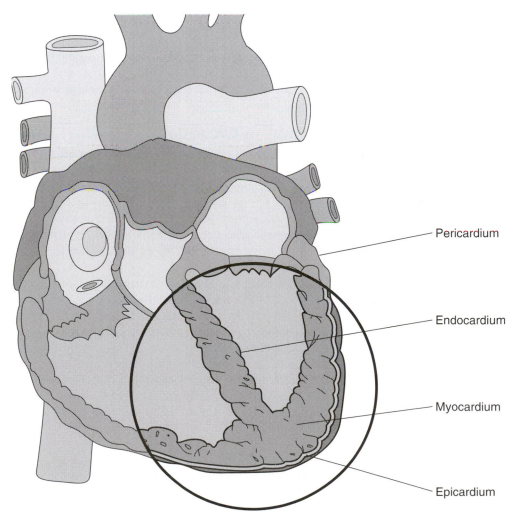

Figure 1-3   Heart muscle layers

■ **myocardium:** *middle layer of heart muscle, responsible for pumping action*

■ **epicardium:** *external layer of the heart and part of pericardial sac*

■ **Purkinje fibers:** *modified myocardial cells found in distal areas of the bundle branches*

■ **pericardium:** *double-walled, membranous sac enclosing the heart*

Myocardium

Myocardial cells form the middle layer of cardiac muscle. These muscle cells coordinate contraction and cause the chambers of the heart to contract and pump blood. Myocardium is thin in the atria, thicker in the right ventricle, and thickest in the left ventricle.

Epicardium

The epicardium, a fatty layer on the outer surface of the myocardium, forms the protective covering of the heart. The outermost epicardial layers, the **peri-cardium,** consist of two layers with a small amount of lubricating fluid between them. This pericardial sac encloses the entire heart, holds it in place, and reduces friction as the heart beats.

Clinical application: Pericarditis, myocarditis, and epicarditis are inflammations of these heart layers. Myocardial infarction is the result of dead tissue areas in the myocardium caused by interruption of blood supply to this area.

▨▨▨ PHYSIOLOGY OF CIRCULATION

Pulmonary, Systemic, and Coronary Circulations

In addition to pumping blood for circulation, the heart contracts to produce a pressure that forces blood to flow through the blood vessels to supply nutrients to the body cells and to remove wastes. The blood vessels of the cardiovascular system divide into two major pathways—the **pulmonary circulation** and the **systemic circulation** (Figure 1-4). The systemic circuit consists of blood vessels to transport oxygenated blood from the heart to all parts of the body and back again; the pulmonary circuit is responsible for carrying deoxygenated blood from the right ventricle of the heart to the lungs and back to the heart. Although the blood flowing through the heart chambers nourishes all the tissues of the body, it does not nourish the heart muscle itself. The right and left coronary arteries supply the **coronary circulation** to the heart muscle (Figure 1-5).

■ **pulmonary circulation:** *flow of blood from right ventricle to lungs, where carbon dioxide is exchanged for oxygen and returned to the left atrium*

■ **systemic circulation:** *flow of oxygen-rich blood to all body tissue and organs from the left ventricle via the arteries and its return to the right atrium via the veins*

■ **coronary circulation:** *blood supply to the myocardium of the heart from branches of the aorta*

Pathway of Circulation

Blood depleted of its oxygen flows from all tissues of the body via the systemic circulation into the right atrium. Blood in the right atrium passes into the right ventricle. Contraction of the right ventricle pushes blood against the tricuspid valve, forcing it closed; and against the pulmonary semilunar valve, forcing it open and allowing blood to enter the pulmonary artery. The pulmonary artery carries the blood to the lungs where carbon dioxide is released from the blood for expiration by the lungs and exchanged for oxygen (Figure 1-6).

Blood from the lungs, entering the left atrium through four pulmonary veins, passes through the mitral valve into the left ventricle. Contraction of the left ventricle pushes blood against the mitral valve, forcing it closed; and against the aortic valve, opening it and permitting blood to enter the aorta. From the aorta, the arteries transport the oxygen-rich, bright-red blood to the body. Individual cells exchange the oxygen for carbon dioxide and other wastes. Oxygen-depleted, almost purple-tinted blood returns to the right side of the heart through the veins. The right heart then pumps blood to the lungs again. The entire process is repeated between 60 to 100 times per minute in the normal individual at rest.

Cardiac Cycle

■ **cardiac cycle:** *rhythmic repetition of the mechanical and electrical events that constitute the heartbeat*

The **cardiac cycle** is the series of events constituting a complete heartbeat. Heart action regulates contraction of the atrial walls while the ventricular walls

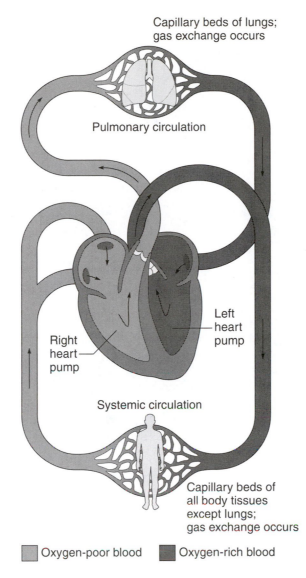

Capillary beds of lungs;
gas exchange occurs

Pulmonary circulation

Left heart pump

Right heart pump

Systemic circulation

Capillary beds of all body tissues except lungs; gas exchange occurs

Oxygen-poor blood   Oxygen-rich blood

Figure 1-4 Systemic and pulmonary circulations

■ **systole:** *period in which the mechanical and electrical events of the heart are active. Mechanical systole is characterized by contraction; electrical systole involves depolarization*

■ **diastole:** *period in which the mechanical and electrical events of the heart are relaxed. Mechanical diastole is relaxation; electrical diastole involves repolarization*

relax; ventricular walls contract while the atrial walls relax. The atria and ventricles remain relaxed at the end of each cardiac cycle for only a moment before the entire cycle is repeated. This contraction and pushing of blood out to the body is known as **systole** or the systolic phase of the cardiac cycle. Relaxation of the heart, allowing expansion and refilling of the chambers, is considered to be **diastole** or the diastolic phase of the cardiac cycle (Figure 1-7).

Systole and Diastole

The cycle of a heartbeat proceeds through these stages:

Atrial systole—Ventricles acquire blood as the atria contract.

Ventricular systole—Contraction of the ventricles forces blood out the pulmonary artery and aorta.

Atrial diastole—The atria begin refilling during ventricular systole.

Ventricular diastole—Blood from the atria begins refilling the ventricles during atrial systole.

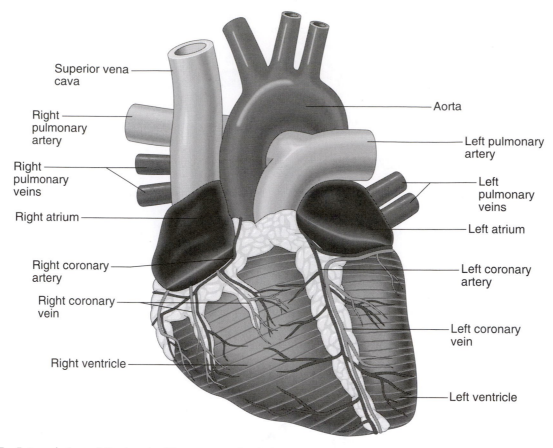

Figure 1-5   External view of the heart with coronary circulation

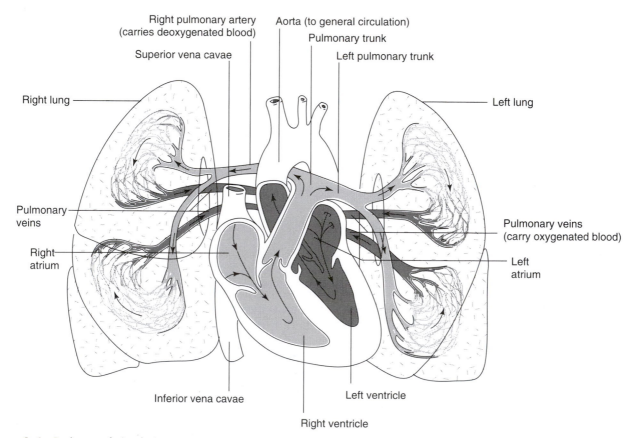

Figure 1-6   Pathway of circulation

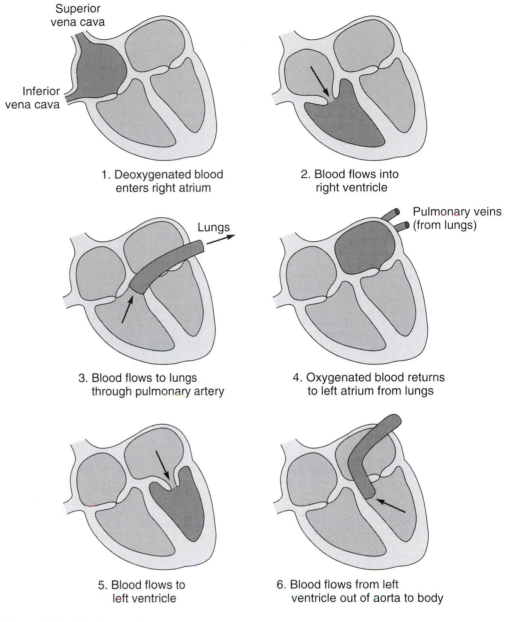

Superior
vena cava

Inferior
vena cava

1. Deoxygenated blood
enters right atrium

2. Blood flows into
right ventricle

Lungs

3. Blood flows to lungs
through pulmonary artery

Pulmonary veins
(from lungs)

4. Oxygenated blood returns
to left atrium from lungs

5. Blood flows to
left ventricle

6. Blood flows from left
ventricle out of aorta to body

Figure 1-7   Cardiac cycle

▬▬ CONDUCTION PATHWAYS OF THE HEART

A network of conducting tissue within the heart actually initiates each heartbeat and controls rhythm. Throughout the myocardium are specialized cardiac muscle tissues that do not contract; instead, they initiate and distribute cardiac impulses throughout the myocardium (Figure 1-8).

Sinoatrial Node

■ *sinoatrial (SA) node:*
natural pacemaker of the heart, positioned in the right atrium

A tiny bundle of nerve tissue in the right atrium, the **sinoatrial (SA) node,** begins the electrical wave that starts the heartbeat. The SA node is the main cardiac pacemaker from which wave-like impulses are relayed through the atrium. The membranes of the nodal cells, which lie in close proximity to each other, can excite themselves without being stimulated by nerve fibers. These impulses spread rhythmically into the surrounding myocardium and stimulate cardiac muscle fibers to contract. The right atrium is stimulated slightly before the left atrium. Electrical impulses are generated by the SA node at the rate of 60 to 100 times per minute.

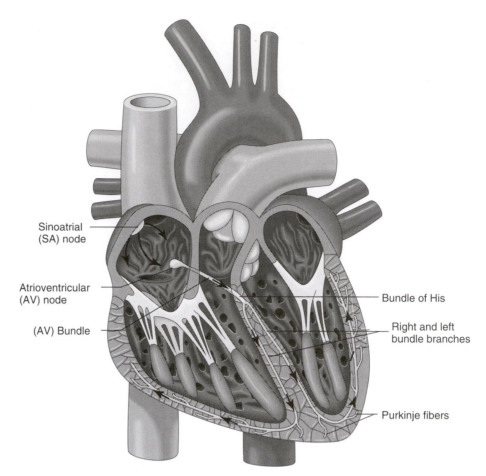

Sinoatrial
(SA) node

Atrioventricular
(AV) node

(AV) Bundle

Bundle of His

Right and left
bundle branches

Purkinje fibers

Figure 1-8   The heartbeat is controlled by electrical impulses.

Atrioventricular Node

As soon as the atria are stimulated, part of the electrical impulse travels via internodal tracts to a connecting mass of specialized muscle tissue. The **atrioventricular (AV) node** lies on the floor of the right atrium near the portion of the septum separating the atria and just above the ventricles. These smaller fibers of the AV node cause a delay in the impulse. Two basic functions of the AV node include: (1) protecting the ventricles from excessively fast heart rates that may originate in the atrium and (2) serving as a pacemaker for the heart should the SA node fail. The AV node will initiate impulses at the rate of 40 to 60 times per minute.

AV Bundle (Bundle of His)

The wave of excitation spreads to fibers known as the **AV bundle (bundle of His)**, which is next to and contiguous with the AV node. As the impulse reaches the interventricular septum, the pathway divides into the right and left bundle branches.

Bundle Branches

The right **bundle branch** extends along the right side of the septum and reaches the base of the right ventricle, where it divides into a network supplying the myocardium of the right ventricle. The left bundle branch extends along the left side of the septum and divides into anterior and posterior segments. The anterior division supplies the upper portion of the left ventricle; the posterior division supplies the lower portion.

■ *atrioventricular (AV) node:* pacemaking cells found in right atrium on interatrial septum

■ *AV bundle (bundle of His):* fibers within the interventricular septum that carry impulses to the bundle branches located in the right and left ventricles

■ *bundle branches:* groups of Purkinje fibers, arising from the bundle of His, that conduct electrical impulses to the right and left ventricles

Purkinje Fibers

Halfway down the septum, the right bundle branch and both segments of the left bundle branch give rise to a complex network of enlarged Purkinje fibers. These fibers spread extensively along the septum, continuing downward to the apex of the heart, where they curve around the tips of the ventricles and upward over the lateral walls of the ventricular chambers. Although initiating impulses at the rate of only 20 to 40 times per minute, the ventricles may also function as a backup system for pacemaking if required by the heart. The bundle of His, the right and left bundle branches, and the Purkinje fibers are responsible for contracting the ventricles.

▓▓▓▓ ELECTROPHYSIOLOGY OF THE HEART

Special Properties of Cardiac Cells

Cardiac cells exhibit four unique properties:

- automaticity
- excitability
- conductivity
- contractility

Automaticity is the inherent ability of certain myocardial cells to initiate and maintain rhythmic heart activity without the assistance of a neurological supply. The SA node contains the pacemaking cells with the highest degree of automaticity and the most rapid discharge rate. *Excitability* is the inherent ability of both pacemaking cells and non-pacemaking myocardial cells to respond to an impulse or stimulus. *Conductivity* allows the myocardial cell to relay an impulse to a neighboring cell. This impulse has the potential to create a wave of excitation that propagates throughout the entire tissue. *Contractility* is the ability to respond to an electrical impulse with pumping action.

Electrical Activity of the Heart

There are two basic types of myocardial cells: those capable of contractility and those capable of conduction. The working myocardial cells, containing contractile proteins with the ability to shorten and then return to their original length, produce the mechanical pumping action of the heart. Timing and synchronizing the contractile cells is the responsibility of the pacemaking network of the electrical conduction cells of the myocardium. Generated impulses create a rhythmic repetition of beats called *cardiac cycles*. Each cardiac cycle consists of electrical and mechanical activation (systole) and recovery (diastole). A brief delay occurs before the onset of electrical and mechanical diastole because the mechanical events are initiated by the electrical events (Figure 1-9).

Contraction of the Heart

Cardiac cells polarize electrically in their resting state. In this resting state, the cell has a positive charge on the outside of the cell membrane and a negative charge on the inside of the cell. Membrane pumps maintain the electrical polarity of the cell by ensuring the appropriate distribution of the primary ions: potassium, sodium, chloride, and calcium. In this way they keep the negative charge inside the cell membrane.

Depolarization of the Cell

For contraction to occur, the cell membrane must be electrically activated. The process of **depolarization** causes a change in the properties of the cell as the result of the flow across the cell membrane of positive ions into the cell and of negative ions to the outside of the cell membrane. Depolarization is the fundamental electrical event of the heart. This wave of depolarization, representing a

■ *depolarization: process in which there is minimal difference in electrical charge between the inside of a cell and the outside of the cell*

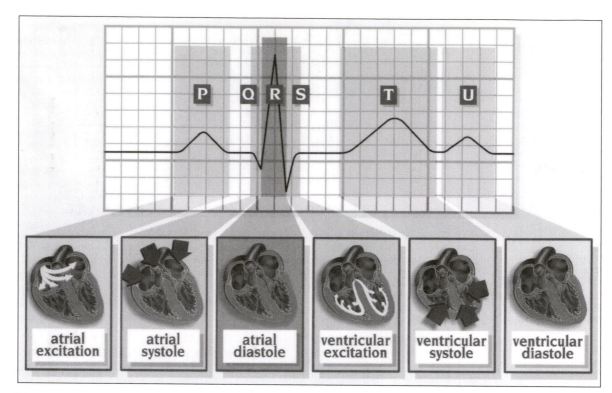

Figure 1-9   Electrical and mechanical events. (Copyright Marquette Electronics, Marquette, Wisconsin)

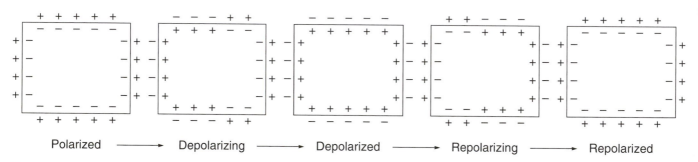

Polarized ——→ Depolarizing ——→ Depolarized ——→ Repolarizing ——→ Repolarized

Figure 1-10   Depolarization and repolarization of cell

flow of electricity, propagates from cell to cell across the entire heart (Figure 1-10). This electrical impulse is transmitted to the chest wall, where it may be detected and recorded as an ECG.

Repolarization

■ **repolarization:** condition or state in which the inside of the cell is considerably more positive than the outside of the cell

Relaxation (resting state) after contraction occurs by a process called **repolarization,** in which the polarity returns negative ions to the inside of the cell and positive ions to the outside of the cell. After depolarization is complete, the cardiac cells restore their resting polarity through repolarization (Figure 1-10). Table 1-1 shows the relationship between the electrical and mechanical actions in the cardiac cycle.

The waves of depolarization and repolarization represent electrical activity that is capable of detection. Electrodes placed on the surface of the body sense this activity, which is recorded by the ECG machine and displayed graphically as an ECG (Figure 1-11). The different waves, segments, intervals, and complexes displayed as the ECG are manifestations of the two processes of depolarization and repolarization by the myocardial cells of the heart.

Table 1-1 Cardiac Cycle Terminology

	Systole	Diastole
Electrical Cycle	Depolarization	Repolarization
	Activation	Recovery
	Excitation	Recovery
Mechanical Cycle	Contraction	Relaxation
	Emptying	Filling
	Shortening	Lengthening

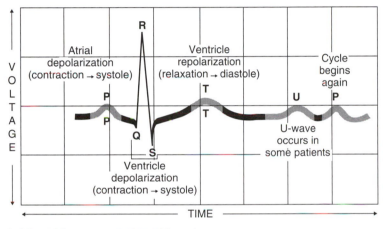

Q wave is a negative deflection or wave.

R wave is a positive deflection or wave.

S wave is a negative wave.

T wave is a positive wave and represents ventricular repolarization.

U wave (occasionally seen in some patients) is a positive deflection and associated with repolarization.

Figure 1-11   ECG representation of heartbeat

REVIEW QUESTIONS

Multiple Choice Questions

1. The heart muscle receives its blood supply from the:
   a. pulmonary circulation.
   b. systemic circulation.
   c. aorta.
   d. coronary circulation.

2. The left ventricle:
   a. pumps blood to the lungs.
   b. receives oxygenated blood from the lungs.
   c. pumps blood to all parts of the body except the lungs.
   d. receives deoxygenated blood.

3. The endocardium is the:
   a. inner layer of cardiac muscle cells.
   b. middle layer of heart muscle.
   c. external layer of the heart and part of the pericardial sac.
   d. upper, collecting chamber of the heart.

4. The atrioventricular (AV) node is:
   a. found within the interventricular septum.
   b. the natural pacemaker of the heart.
   c. found in the right atrium on the interatrial septum.
   d. located within the network of the Purkinje fibers.

5. Depolarization is:
   a. mechanical diastole.
   b. the condition in which the inside of the myocardial cell is considerably more positive in relation to the outside of the cell.
   c. rhythmic repetition of heartbeats.
   d. electrical systole.

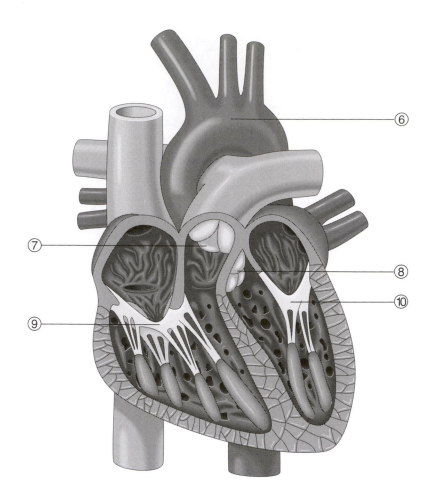

Matching Questions

Fill in the correct name for the numbered areas shown in the accompanying figure.

6. _____

7. _____

8. _____

9. _____

10. _____

Match each term with the letter of the correct definition.

11. chordae tendineae:

12. pericardium:

13. sinoatrial (SA) node:

14. pulmonary semilunar valve:

15. myocardium:

    a. double-walled, membranous sac enclosing the heart

    b. heart valve between the right ventricle and the pulmonary artery

    c. natural pacemaker of the heart, positioned in the right atrium

    d. strong, fibrous strings attached to cardiac valves

    e. middle layer of heart muscle

Short Answer/Fill in the Blank

16. Myocardial cells are charged or _____ in their resting state.

17. The electrical cycle of the heartbeat begins at the _____ .

18. The pacemaker of the heart is located in the _____ .

19. Conduction proceeds to the _____ .

20. The wave of excitation spreads to the _____ which is contiguous to the AV node.

21. Cardiac cells exhibit four unique properties:

    a. _____

    b. _____

    c. _____

    d. _____

The Normal Electrocardiogram

OBJECTIVES:

After reading this chapter, you will be able to:

Explain how electrical current in the heart is generated.

Differentiate between ECG waves, segments, intervals, and complexes.

Describe how the movement of electricity through the heart produces predictable wave patterns.

Describe the method of detection and recording of these wave patterns by the ECG machine.

OVERVIEW

After invention of the ECG machine by Einthoven, the heart of a patient could be monitored by electrodes placed on the skin. Electrode pads sense the electrical conduction of the myocardial cells throughout the heart. The electrode sensors attach by cables or lead wires to an ECG module. The activating electrical wave, which travels across the atria, down the AV node, and through the ventricles, can then easily be measured and graphically recorded. If the patient is lying quietly, the only significant muscle-electrical activity in the body is the heartbeat. A recording device is able to tune in on this electrical field.

DETECTION AND RECORDING METHODS

All human cells are electrically charged with more positively charged particles on the outer surface of the cell membrane than on the inner surface. These charged particles are called *ions*. The difference between the ions inside the cell and outside the cell results in the electrical **transmembrane potential** of the cell membrane. The transmembrane potential or resting membrane state is the beginning of the **action potential,** which is the positive electrical potential recorded from within a cell. The action potential includes the changes during the process of depolarization and repolarization within a cell as it is activated by an electrical current or impulse.

Depolarization reverses the charge on the cell membrane, making the cell membrane electrically negative as compared to the inside of the cell. Repolarization returns the positive charge on the cell membrane. Repolarization has four phases that delay the impulse so that repolarization is not too rapid. If cardiac cells repolarized rapidly, they would be ready too soon to conduct another impulse, and unable to conduct impulses in a coordinated fashion.

Because cardiac muscle fibers are interconnected, action potentials are propagated and moved from depolarized cells to adjoining polarized cells. The **refractory period** is the time during which the cell is unable to respond to a stimulus or conduct an impulse. Before cells can conduct the next electrical stimulus, they must return to their polarized state. The depolarization-repolarization cycle is depicted by the ECG.

■ **transmembrane potential:** *the electrical difference between the inside of the cell and the outside of the cell*

■ **action potential:** *the changes during the process of depolarization and repolarization within a cell as it is activated by an electrical impulse*

■ **refractory period:** *time during which the cell is unable to respond to a stimulus*

■ *vector: path of impulse displaying the direction and magnitude of the electrical current*

The path the action potential, or impulse, takes as it spreads through the myocardium is represented by a current or **vector.** Arrows represent vectors and display the direction and magnitude of the current. The action potential spreads throughout the myocardium in a sequential manner. Not all cells in the myocardium are depolarized at the same time. Current moves from depolarized (negatively charged) cells to polarized (positively charged) cells as the impulse moves from the base (atria) to the apex (ventricles) of the heart.

In the healthy heart, the movement of current (vectors) proceeds in the same sequence during each cardiac cycle. Each myocardial cell forms an instant or discrete vector within the heart. The net size and direction of multiple forces may be added and subtracted to determine the vector. The sum of all the instant vectors is the mean vector or the ECG. The heart maintains a rhythmic, pumping action as a result of the electrical impulses generated and transmitted throughout the electrical conduction system of the heart. The conduction system transmits electrical impulses from cell to cell throughout the heart along the conduction pathway previously discussed.

Cardiac cells transfer the electrical impulse to other cardiac cells with exceptional speed, making it appear as if the cells are responding simultaneously. The transmission speed of impulse propagation varies from site to site within the heart (see Table 2-1).

ECG Machine

■ *galvanometer: the early ECG machine*

■ *electrodes: small, specially prepared tabs with conductive gel placed in direct contact with the skin to detect electrical current from within the heart*

■ *stylus: the writing arm or point of the ECG machine*

An ECG machine consists of a writing arm, a **galvanometer** (or recording device), lead wires, and **electrodes.** A galvanometer is a current meter connected to a **stylus** needle, which responds by heat or pressure either upward or downward in direction and magnitude according to the current flowing through the meter. Small electrode tabs placed on the patient provide direct contact with the skin and transmit electrical current from the body. The electrodes are attached by lead wires to the recording device in an arrangement of two or more electrodes per lead.

As a depolarization or vector moves toward a negative electrode, it produces a downward or negative deflection on the ECG. When the depolarization moves toward a positive electrode, it produces an upward or positive deflection on the ECG (Figure 2-1). The ECG is a tracing of electrical voltage produced by the continual depolarization and repolarization of the myocardium. The stylus of the ECG machine remains at the zero, or isoelectric, baseline and records a straight line if not deflected upward or downward. At baseline, the current is absent or too weak to move the recording device. A flow of electrical current that causes a deflection (movement) of the point of the stylus also causes the stylus to inscribe a wave on the ECG paper.

The ECG machine shows direction and magnitude of the electrical current produced by the heart. At any point during depolarization or repolarization, the current is flowing in a multitude of directions. The ECG machine responds to the resultant forces at each moment in time to draw a single straight line. The

Table 2-1 Transmission Speeds	
AV node	200 mm/second
Ventricular muscle	400 mm/second
Atrial muscle	1,000 mm/second
Purkinje system	4,000 mm/second

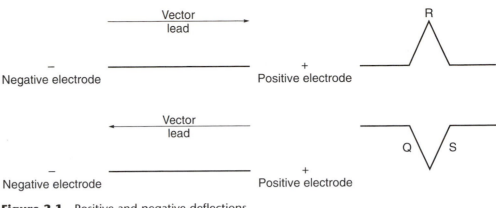

Figure 2-1   Positive and negative deflections

ECG machine is able to resolve all the individual forces into a resultant force with direction and magnitude.

Waves, Segments, Intervals, and Complexes

Deflections from the baseline are called **waves** and are designated P, QRS, and T. **Segments** or straight lines are the spaces created between the waves. **Intervals** consist of a wave and a connecting straight line and are designated at the beginning and end of their associated waves. **Complexes** are groups of related recorded waves.

Clinical application: The **ST segment** is the space between the S wave and the T wave. This segment is measured from the end of the S wave to the beginning of the T wave. Interval measurement is calculated from the beginning of the first wave. The **QT interval** is from the start of the Q wave to the end of the T wave.

The initial wave of a cardiac cycle represents depolarization (activation) of the atria electrically and is called the **P wave** (Figure 2-2). The first portion of the P wave denotes right atrial activation or depolarization; the last segment of the P wave represents the completion of left atrial activation. Its midsection represents completion of right atrial activation and initiation of left atrial activation.

AV node activation occurs in the middle of the P wave. The wave representing ventricular depolarization obscures any wave that records electrical recovery of the atria. A pause lasting one-tenth of a second occurs after the impulse reaches the AV node. This pause, which allows the atria to empty before the ventricles contract, separates atrial from ventricular activity. This delay is shown on the ECG as the **P-R interval** (Figure 2-2). A normal P-R interval, the line from the start of atrial depolarization to the start of ventricular depolarization, is the measurement from the onset of the P wave to the beginning of the **QRS complex**, lasting 0.12 to 0.20 seconds.

Clinical application: The P-R interval varies with heart rate, age, and physique. The P-R interval is inversely related to heart rate and directly related to the size of the heart. That is, the greater the heart rate, the shorter the P-R interval; the larger the heart, the larger the P-R interval.

The QRS complex, the next group of recorded waves, represents activation of the ventricles. Because the ventricles are considerably larger than the atria, the amplitude of the QRS is taller than the atrial P wave. After the impulse stimulates the AV node and propagates down the AV bundle into the bundle branches, it transmits to the Purkinje fibers and into the myocardial cells, causing ventricular depolarization. The first downward stroke of the complex is the **Q wave,** followed by the normally upward **R wave.** The Q wave represents activation in the interventricular septum. (The Q wave may be absent.) The R wave, the predominant portion of the QRS complex, is impulse progression through the right and left ventricular myocardium. A negative deflection following an R wave is called an **S wave** and denotes completion of left

---

- **waves:** *deflections from the baseline*
- **segments:** *the straight lines connecting waves*
- **intervals:** *a wave in addition to a connecting straight line*
- **complexes:** *groups of related, recorded waves*
- **ST segment:** *isoelectric line from the end of S wave to the beginning of T wave*
- **QT interval:** *measures beginning of ventricular depolarization to end of ventricular repolarization*
- **P wave:** *records atrial depolarization and contraction*

- **P-R interval:** *time for electrical impulse to conduct through atria and the AV node*
- **QRS complex:** *represents depolarization or contraction of the ventricles*

- **Q wave:** *first negative deflection of QRS complex from impulse activation in the interventricular septum*
- **R wave:** *first upward deflection of QRS complex from impulse progression through the ventricles*
- **S wave:** *a negative deflection denoting completion of left ventricular activation*

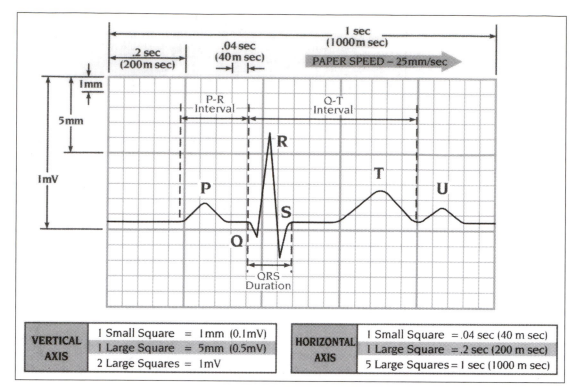

Figure 2-2   The ECG configuration. (Copyright Marquette Electronics, Marquette, Wisconsin)

ventricular activation. The normal duration of the QRS complex, 0.04 to 0.10 seconds, indicates the time of ventricular depolarization.

Besides the depolarization wave, a wave of repolarization also exists. Repolarization of the ventricles, the **T wave,** occurs so that the myocardial cells may regain their negative charge and depolarize again. The wave of atrial repolarization coincides with ventricular depolarization but is obscured by the more prominent QRS complex.

The ST segment, an isoelectric (flat) line having no voltage from the end of the S wave to the beginning of the T wave, is a pause after ventricular depolarization. The QT interval, measured from the onset of the Q wave to completion of the T wave, measures the time from the beginning of ventricular depolarization to the end of ventricular repolarization. The duration is 0.35 to 0.45 seconds.

■ **T wave:** *represents repolarization (relaxing) of ventricles*

▓▓ **EXPLANATION OF ECG PAPER**

Time and Voltage

Because the ECG displays the amount of electrical activity generated by the heart and the time required for those generated electrical impulses to travel throughout the heart during a heartbeat, the ECG is recorded on a graph/grid that is one millimeter long and one millimeter high. A darker line occurs every five millimeters. The height and depth of a wave are measured in millimeters. The vertical axis displays voltage with the distance along each small square equal to one millivolt (mV); each large square is 5×0.1 mV $= 0.5$ mV. The horizontal axis represents time. Each small square is 0.04 seconds in time (one small square is 1 mm in length); each large square is 5×0.04 seconds $= 0.20$ seconds in time (each large square is 5 mm in length). The duration of any part of the cardiac cycle may be determined by measuring along the horizontal axis (Figure 2-3).

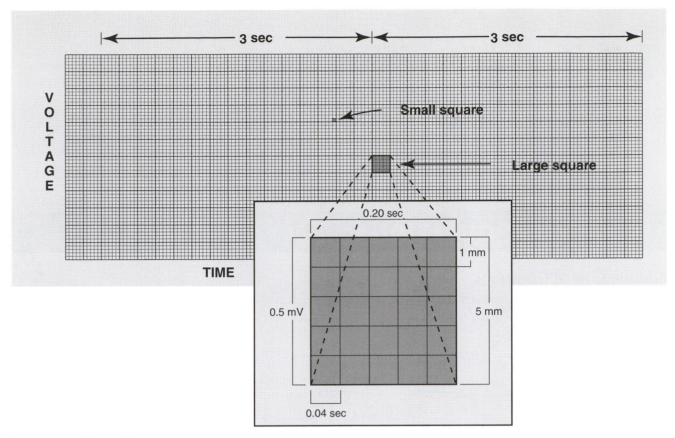

Figure 2-3 ECG graph paper

Clinical application: If the heart is normal, each cardiac cycle will require approximately 0.8 seconds of time. Each wave of the cardiac cycle (P, QRS, and T) may be examined and measured (according to size, shape, and location on the ECG) by a physician for determination of overall cardiac health.

Clinical application: ECG paper rolls out of the ECG machine at a preset speed of 25 mm per second. Pediatric ECGs use a preset speed of 50 mm per second, because of the faster heart rates of infants and young children.

HEART RATE CALCULATION

To determine the rhythm of the heart, the first step is to calculate the heart rate. Many ECG machines display the heart rate with the printed ECG. Special rate rulers for measuring also exist. Because each P, QRS, and T wave cycle represents a heartbeat, and time is measured on the horizontal axis, heart rate may be manually calculated from the ECG tracing. Count the number of large squares (5 small squares or 200 msec) between R waves and divide into 300. For example, if there are 6 large squares between R waves, the heart rate is 50 beats per minute.

NORMAL AND ABNORMAL RHYTHM IDENTIFICATION

Sinus rhythms originate in the SA node, the pacemaker of the heart. In sinus rhythms, all P waves appear like other P waves; QRS complexes resemble each other. The P-R interval remains constant throughout the ECG tracing. Sinus rhythm exhibits regular P-P and R-R cycles and regular P-R intervals.

Sinus **bradycardia** occurs when the sinus rate is less than 60 beats per minute. A slower heart rate occurs at rest and in athletic individuals. Most

■ *bradycardia: a heart rhythm less than 60 beats per minute* patients maintain sinus rates between 60 and 100 beats per minute. When exercising, a patient may exhibit a heart rate above 100 beats per minute, which is known as sinus **tachycardia.**

■ **tachycardia:** *a heart rhythm more than 100 beats per minute*

Clinical application: A patient should exhibit an appropriate heart rate under appropriate conditions. A sinus bradycardia rhythm when exercising would be inappropriate, as would a sinus tachycardia rhythm while sleeping.

Atrial rhythm is regular when the distance between P waves remains constant; ventricular rhythm is regular when the distance between R waves is constant throughout the ECG recording. Otherwise the rhythms are called *irregular* or *arrhythmias.*

REVIEW QUESTIONS

Multiple Choice Questions

1. The QRS complex is representative of:
   a. ventricular repolarization.
   b. atrial depolarization.
   c. ventricular depolarization.
   d. atrial repolarization

2. The wave that represents electrical impulses spreading through the atria is the:
   a. Q wave.
   b. S wave.
   c. T wave.
   d. P wave.

3. Which wave depicts ventricular repolarization on the ECG?
   a. T
   b. P
   c. Q
   d. S

4. If electrical current flows _____ the recording electrode, the deflection is _____, so that an upright wave is recorded.
   a. away from, positive
   b. toward, negative
   c. away from, negative
   d. toward, positive

5. The P-R interval is measured from the _____ of the P wave to the _____ of the QRS complex.
   a. onset, end
   b. onset, beginning
   c. end, end
   d. end, beginning

Matching Questions

Fill in the correct names for the numbered areas shown in the accompanying figure.

6. _____

7. _____

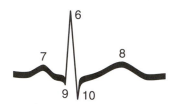

8. _____

9. _____

10. _____

Match each term with the letter of the correct definition.

11. complex _____

12. P-R interval _____

13. R wave _____

14. ST segment _____

15. P wave _____

16. waves _____

17. Q wave _____

18. intervals _____

19. S _____

20. segment _____
   a. first negative deflection of QRS complex
   b. negative deflection denoting completion of left ventricle activation
   c. isoelectric line from end of S wave to beginning of T wave
   d. deflections from baseline
   e. groups of related, recorded waves
   f. time for impulses to conduct through atria and AV node
   g. first upward deflection of QRS complex
   h. a wave plus a connecting, straight line
   i. straight lines connecting waves
   j. records atrial depolarization and contraction

Lead Systems

OBJECTIVES:

After reading this chapter, you will be able to:

- Describe the purpose of an ECG lead.
- Differentiate between unipolar and bipolar leads.
- Describe the orientation of all 12 leads.
- Explain chest and limb lead placement.

OVERVIEW

Each ECG lead views the heart at a unique angle along 12 different paths. Every lead consists of a positive pole and a negative pole and measures the electrical difference between the poles. Einthoven's triangle represents the location of these positive and negative electrodes or poles as equal distances from the heart. Limb leads measure the electrical difference between two electrodes on the frontal plane of the chest. Bipolar limb leads compare electrical potentials between two sites on the chest. Unipolar limb leads use the extremities as the positive pole and the negative pole as the center of the Einthoven triangle. Each electrode records from a different angle and is a unique view of the same cardiac activity. The waves from each lead appear slightly different because the electrical activity is monitored from slightly different positions. Together the limb and chest leads provide overlapping views of cardiac activity.

PRINCIPLES OF EINTHOVEN'S TRIANGLE

Initially Einthoven arranged recording electrodes on the right and left arms and left leg, with an additional grounding electrode on the right leg. Wires or **leads** attach to the sensing electrodes. Each lead measures the electrical difference between the two electrodes (poles); one lead is negative and the other is positive. **Einthoven's triangle** displays the position of the negative and positive electrodes (poles) as equidistant from the heart (Figure 3-1).

■ **leads:** long, coated electrical wires which are part of the apparatus that measures electrical differences between electrodes

■ **Einthoven's triangle:** equilateral triangle composed of the limb leads I, II and III; provides information from the frontal plane of the chest

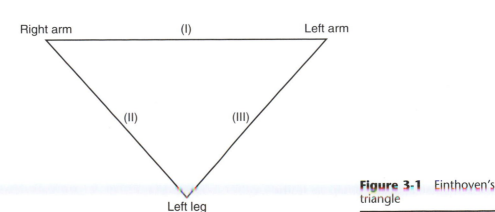

Figure 3-1 Einthoven's triangle

Because the heart is a three-dimensional organ, its electrical activity must be assessed in three dimensions also. As Einthoven and early electrocardiographers discovered, the heart could not adequately be analyzed using only the three limb electrodes. With those three limb electrodes, electrical activity was appraised from base to apex and from the left to the right side of the heart. Today, 12 other viewpoints are used for electrical analysis.

TWELVE PERSPECTIVES OF THE HEART

The standard ECG uses 12 leads. Each lead is determined by the placement and location of the electrodes on the patient. Each view is a function of the electrical potential difference between a positive and a negative body surface electrode. Six of these leads provide frontal plane views of the heart and six show the horizontal or transverse plane.

LIMB LEADS

The electrodes placed on the arms and legs of the patient form the basis for the **limb leads** (Figure 3-2). Limb leads reflect the impulses moving in electrical currents in the vertical plane or **frontal plane.** The frontal plane mirrors the waves of depolarization and repolarization moving up and down and right and left. The six limb leads include the three standard leads, I, II and III, and the three augmented leads, AVR, AVL, and AVF.

The standard limb leads, also known as **bipolar leads,** form a pair of limb electrodes, one becoming the positive pole and the other the negative pole. A bipolar lead reflects the difference in electrical potential between the two connected limb electrodes. The right arm electrode is the negative pole and the left arm electrode is the positive pole in lead I. Lead II uses the left leg electrode as the positive pole and the right arm as the negative pole. Lead III has the negative pole on the left arm and the positive pole on the left leg. Leads I, II, and III compose the Einthoven triangle.

A **hexaxial reference system,** formed by the intersection of leads I, II, and III near the center of the ventricles, is known as the **central terminal.** The leads formed by this intersection—AVR, AVL, and AVF—use the central terminal as the negative pole and the limb electrodes as positive poles (Figure 3-3). In these **unipolar leads,** the central terminal has zero potential. Unipolar limb leads measure the absolute force at the site of a positive electrode. AVR, AVL, and AVF function as unipolar leads. A mechanism built into the ECG machine combines the negative electrodes of the three lead wires on the extremities into one common electrode. Although electrodes are placed on all extremities, the right leg electrode functions as a ground. AVR, AVL, and AVF display the absolute elec-

- **limb leads:** *sensing electrodes placed on the wrists and ankles to view electrical impulses in the frontal plane*
- **frontal plane:** *a vertical position of the body lying perpendicular to the horizontal level*
- **bipolar leads:** *leads composed of a negative and a positive pole; reflect the difference in electrical potential between the two*
- **hexaxial reference system:** *formation of six segments revolving around a central axis or point*
- **central terminal:** *the combination of all three limb electrodes serving as the negative pole to form a V lead*
- **unipolar leads:** *measure absolute electrical force at the site of a positive electrode*

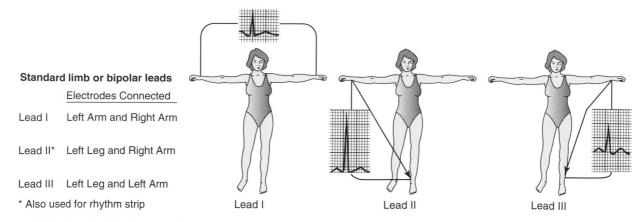

Standard limb or bipolar leads

	Electrodes Connected
Lead I	Left Arm and Right Arm
Lead II*	Left Leg and Right Arm
Lead III	Left Leg and Left Arm

* Also used for rhythm strip

Lead I   Lead II   Lead III

Figure 3-2   Standard limb or bipolar leads

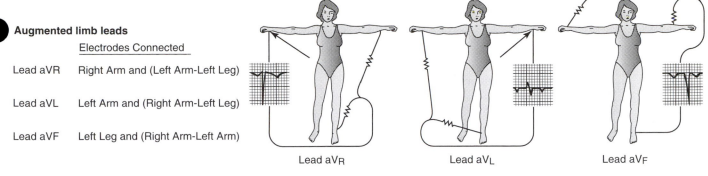

Augmented limb leads

	Electrodes Connected
Lead aVR	Right Arm and (Left Arm-Left Leg)
Lead aVL	Left Arm and (Right Arm-Left Leg)
Lead aVF	Left Leg and (Right Arm-Left Arm)

Lead aV$_R$ Lead aV$_L$ Lead aV$_F$

Figure 3-3   Augmented limb leads

Precordial or chest leads

	Electrodes connected	Placement
V$_1$	V$_1$ and (Left Arm-Right Arm-Left Leg)	Fourth intercostal space at right margin of sternum
V$_2$	V$_2$ and (Left Arm-Right Arm-Left Leg)	Fourth intercostal space at left margin of sternum
V$_4$	V$_4$ and (Left Arm-Right Arm-Left Leg)	Fifth intercostal space at junction of left midclavicular line
V$_3$	V$_3$ and (Left Arm-Right Arm-Left Leg)	Midway between position 2 and position 4
V$_5$	V$_5$ and (Left Arm-Right Arm-Left Leg)	At horizontal level of position 4 at left anterior axillary line
V$_6$	V$_6$ and (Left Arm-Right Arm-Left Leg)	At horizontal level of position 4 at left midaxillary line

Precordial leads

V$_6$
V$_5$
V$_1$ V$_2$ V$_3$ V$_4$

Figure 3-4   Precordial or chest leads

■ *augmented leads: leads that amplify electrical signals*

trical force at the site of each positive limb electrode. VL is the lead designated from the central terminal to the left arm; VR is the lead to the right arm; VF is the lead to the foot. These unipolar leads are also called **augmented leads,** because the electrical signals are so small and far away from the heart that they must be amplified by the ECG machine. The amplified signals increase the size of the electrical action potentials by 50% without a change in the configuration of the electrode.

CHEST LEADS

■ *precordial leads: leads situated on the chest directly overlying the heart*

The six chest leads, or **precordial leads,** demonstrate electrical forces moving anteriorly and posteriorly in a transverse plane. Although the chest leads are unipolar leads, they do not have to be augmented, because the precordial leads lie in close proximity to the heart. Each chest lead senses the myocardial activity nearest it and records the charges as seen from its point of view. The precordial leads are formed with the central terminal as the negative pole and each chest electrode as the positive pole.

Chest leads, numbered V1 through V6, move from the right to the left side of the heart in successive steps (Figure 3-4). Leads V1 and V2 are placed over the right ventricle; V3 and V4 are positioned over the interventricular septum; V5 and V6 are arranged over the left ventricle. The chest leads are placed around the heart in its anatomical position within the chest. The ECG tracing will show progressive changes from V1 to V6.

▰▰ LEAD PLACEMENT

If electrodes are placed less than 12 centimeters (cm) from the electrical center of the heart (the precordial leads), the amplitudes of the wave deflections are influenced by that closeness to the heart. When an electrode is positioned further than 12 cm from the heart (the limb leads), the height of the deflection is not changed significantly. This fact is based on the concept of electrical infinity. Limb leads are not affected by their distance from the heart. According to this principle, an upper extremity electrode may be placed on the wrist, shoulder, or upper chest and a lower extremity electrode may be positioned on the thigh or ankle.

Clinical application: RA and LA are traditionally placed anywhere on the arm; alternate placement to reduce artifact and provide optimal contact is midway between the elbow and shoulder. ▰▰ **Rationale:** *Usually less hair is present on the upper arms, allowing better electrode contact. Less muscle contraction artifact (as a result of finger movement) appears on the ECG if the upper arms are used.* ▰▰

RL and LL are traditionally positioned a few inches above the ankle; an alternate position to reduce muscle artifact is on the upper leg, as close to the torso as possible. Although alternate locations for limb electrode placement are used by different clinicians and ECG equipment manufacturers, it is recommended that all limb electrodes be positioned using the same method consistently at a facility.

Precordial lead sites are as follows:

- V1 is on the right sternal border in the fourth intercostal space (Figure 3-5).
- V2 is on the left sternal border in the fourth intercostal space.
- V3 is midway between the second and fourth V leads.
- V4 is in the fifth intercostal space measured straight down from the midclavicular notch.

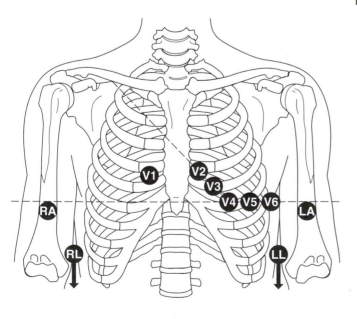

Lead	Electrode location
V1	Fourth intercostal space at the right border of the sternum.
V2	Fourth intercostal space at the left border of the sternum.
V3	Midway between locations V2 and V4.
V4	At the mid-clavicular line in the fifth intercostal space.
V5	At the anterior axillary line on the same horizontal level as V4.
V6	At the mid-axillary line on the same horizontal level as V4 and V5.
RA and LA	Traditionally placed anywhere on the arm, alternate placement to reduce muscle artifact is midway between the elbow and the shoulder.
RL and LL	Traditionally placed a few inches above the ankle, alternate placement to reduce muscle artifact is on the upper leg as close to the torso as possible.

Figure 3-5   Modified Mason-Likar electrode placement. (Copyright Marquette Electronics, Marquette, Wisconsin)

■ V5 is placed between the fourth and sixth V leads at the anterior axillary line.

■ V6 is placed in the fifth intercostal space in the midaxillary level.

Clinical application: ECG electrodes are positioned on the patient according to "anatomical" right and left. This means that right and left are relative to the position of the patient, not the right and left of the health care provider. Right and left are viewed as if the patient were lying in front of you, that is, the right and left of the patient.

Clinical application: When the upper arms and thigh area are used for limb electrode placement, there is not a concern if there is an amputated extremity or a cast is present.

OVERVIEW BY LEAD

Because each electrode records a unique and different view of the same cardiac activity, the deflections on the ECG vary from one electrode to another. Remember that as current flows toward a positive electrode or pole, the ECG waves will be upright or positive. Deflections will be negative when the electrical activity flows toward the negative pole. Therefore, the ECG waves appear differently from various leads, because the electrical activity is monitored from 12 different, specific positions (Figures 3-2, 3-3, and 3-4). Although the electrical activity never changes, the ECG tracing changes slightly in each lead as the angle from which the cardiac activity is monitored changes.

In summary, it is essential to realize that each ECG electrode records only the average current at any given moment. The average current of electrical flow is displayed by a single arrow or vector. At a given instant, this vector is converted by each of the 12 leads into wave patterns as depicted on the ECG (Figure 3-6).

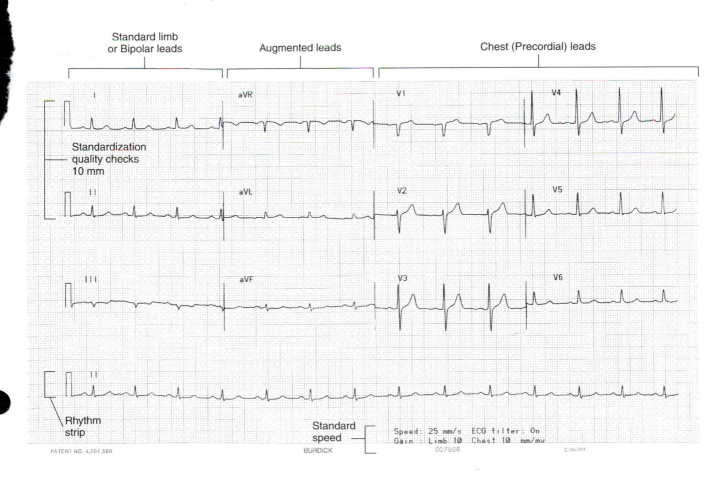

Figure 3-6 12-lead ECG

REVIEW QUESTIONS

Multiple Choice Questions

1. The term *vector* describes the:
   a. negativity of a lead.
   b. direction, magnitude, and sense of an electrical force.
   c. plane of a lead and is represented by an arrow.

2. Augmented leads are:
   a. bipolar and in the horizontal plane.
   b. the same as precordial leads.
   c. unipolar and in the frontal plane.

3. An imaginary electrical center is known as:
   a. the hexaxial system.
   b. the central terminal.
   c. an augmented precordial lead.

4. Unipolar leads:
   a. require amplification.
   b. measure absolute electrical force at the site of a positive electrode.
   c. reflect the difference in electrical potential between a positive pole and a negative pole.

5. Placement of V1 is:
   a. right sternal fourth intercostal space.
   b. left sternal fourth intercostal space.
   c. left sternal fifth intercostal space.

Matching Questions

Fill in the correct names for the numbered areas shown in the accompanying figure.

6. _____

7. _____

8. _____

9. _____

10. _____

11. _____

Match each term with the letter of the correct definition.

12. V1
13. V2
14. V3
15. V4
16. V5
17. V6

a. midway between second and fourth V lead
b. left sternal border between fourth and fifth intercostal space
c. placed in fifth intercostal space in midaxillary level
d. right sternal border between fourth and fifth intercostal space
e. placed in fifth intercostal space measured straight down from the midclavicular notch
f. placed between the fourth and sixth V leads at the anterior axillary line

Short Answer/Fill in the Blank

18. A vertical position of the body lying perpendicular to the horizontal level is the _____ .

19. Six segments revolving around a central axis or point is the _____ system.

20. The _____ leads demonstrate electrical forces moving anteriorly and posteriorly in a transverse plane.

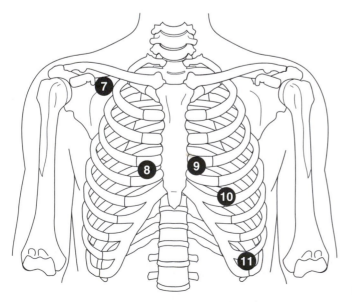

(Copyright Marquette Electronics, Marquette, Wisconsin)

CHAPTER 4

Identifying Rhythms

OBJECTIVES:

After reading this chapter, you will be able to:

Identify normal sinus rhythm.

Differentiate between various sinus rhythms.

Identify and distinguish each atrial arrhythmia.

Compare and contrast atrial and ventricular arrhythmias.

OVERVIEW

Normal electrical conduction pathways of the heart are manifested on the ECG. The usual cardiac rhythm is called normal sinus rhythm. The term *arrhythmia* implies a disturbance in rate, regularity, or site of origin and conduction of the heartbeat. If pacemaking occurs at aberrant (unusual) sites, the conduction alters the P wave and the QRS complex and reflects the change on the ECG. By understanding and comparing basic ECG configurations, simple ECG abnormalities may be recognized. Although rhythm identification is not likely to be the responsibility of the multiskilled health care provider, recognition of potentially fatal arrhythmias by the health care provider, and notification of the nurse and physician so that the patient may be treated, is essential for quality patient care.

ECG CHARACTERISTICS AND CLINICAL SIGNIFICANCE

Recognition of an abnormal ECG tracing is a visual skill perfected by experience and practice. Basic abnormal wave pattern recognition as the ECG is being performed is a responsibility of the health care provider; you must recognize these abnormal patterns if they occur so that a physician may be alerted and the patient treated. Because the ECG records any and all impulses in the heart, it reflects complexes originating from the primary pacemaker sites: the SA node, the AV node, the bundle of His, the right and left bundle branches, and the Purkinje fibers.

The SA node normally sets the heart rate at 60 to 100 beats per minute. Other areas of the heart have the potential to set the heart rate when normal pacemaking fails. These **ectopic** pacemakers usually initiate heart rate only in the presence of disease states or emergency situations. Although all cardiac cells are capable of conducting electrical activity, they usually remain silent unless an aberrant ectopic cell becomes irritable, frustrated, or oxygen-deprived. The ectopic pacemakers exist in all sites of the heart, including the atria, the AV junction, and the ventricles. Ectopic atrial pacemakers initiate pacemaking at a rate of 75 beats per minute; AV junction pacemakers at 40 to 60 beats per minute; ventricular pacemakers at 20 to 40 beats per minute.

When an ectopic beat originates, an unusual-looking complex is recorded on the ECG. Ectopic beats not only look slightly different, but also come at unexpected times. If electrical conduction is altered in any manner within the

■ **ectopic:** *formed in an aberrant (or deviating from the usual) site or focus* chambers of the heart, the P wave or QRS complex will reflect the change. In Chapter 2, we learned that:

■ The P wave represents contraction of the atria.

■ The QRS complex reflects the contraction of the ventricles.

■ The P-R interval measures the time it takes for an electrical impulse to be conducted through the atria and the AV node. The normal P-R interval is 0.12 to 0.20 seconds.

Clinical application: A time faster than 0.12 indicates bypassing of the AV node and a shorter conduction time from the atria to the ventricles. When conduction time is greater than 0.20 seconds, there is slower conduction time from the atria to the ventricles, with the ECG demonstrating AV block.

■ T wave represents the heart relaxing.

■ The ST segment is the time from the end of the QRS complex until the beginning of the T wave.

Rate, regularity, and rhythm are frequently considered together. By comparing cardiac cycles, the rhythm can be characterized as regular or irregular. Normally, the numbers of P waves and QRS complexes are the same. When a constant distance between similar waves exists, the rhythm is regular.

Clinical application: In a clinical situation, Q waves are diagnostic of cardiac myocardial infarction or heart attack. Normal QRS interval is 0.40 to 0.11 seconds; intervals longer than 0.11 seconds reflect abnormal conduction in the ventricles due to blockage of one of the bundle branches. The T wave is a reliable indicator for myocardial ischemia or loss of blood flow to the heart muscle.

SINUS RHYTHM

■ *sinus rhythms:*
heartbeats originating in the SA node

Because electrical conduction pathways normally originate in the SA node, rhythms beginning in the SA node are known as **sinus rhythms.** The P waves and QRS complexes resemble each other. The distance between each P wave (the P to P interval) and the distance between each R wave (the R to R interval) are the same. The following section covers basic wave pattern recognition, as well as a few advanced arrhythmias. New health care providers will be required to recognize certain "lethal" or "panic" waveforms so that they can responsibly inform the registered nurse or physician in charge of a possible medical crisis. Knowledge of the advanced arrhythmias will be invaluable to an ECG monitor tech or an emergency medical technician (EMT).

The following are characteristics of impulses initiated by the SA node and identified as normal sinus rhythm (Figure 4-1).

■ There is a 1:1 relationship between P waves and QRS complexes.

■ P, QRS, and T waves are in appropriate sequential order and of consistent configuration.

■ The P-R interval is 0.12 to 0.20 seconds.

■ The QRS interval is 0.40 to 0.10 seconds.

■ The heart rate is 60 to 100 beats per minute.

■ The P-R interval and atrial and ventricular rhythms are regular.

Dysrhythmias

■ *dysrhythmia*
(arrhythmia): an
abnormality in heart rhythm

The terms **dysrhythmia** and **arrhythmia** are used interchangeably. By definition, *dysrhythmia* is actually an abnormality in rhythm and arrhythmia is indicative of an absence of rhythm. Dysrhythmias are disturbances in impulse formation and/or impulse conduction. Cardiac dysrhythmias occur when there is a:

■ disturbance in automaticity and the rate is too slow or too fast.

■ disturbance in conductivity when the site of impulse formation is not the SA node.

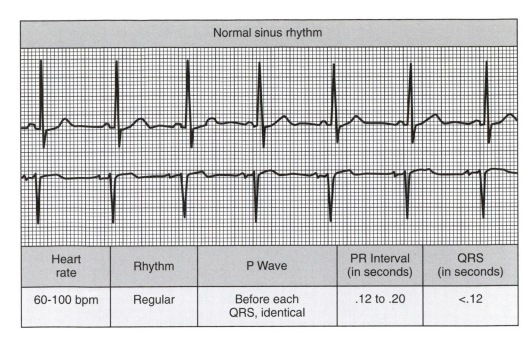

Heart rate	Rhythm	P Wave	PR Interval (in seconds)	QRS (in seconds)
60-100 bpm	Regular	Before each QRS, identical	.12 to .20	<.12

Figure 4-1   Normal sinus rhythm. (Copyright Marquette Electronics, Marquette, Wisconsin)

■ combination of altered automaticity and conductivity and the impulse conduction is abnormal at any point within the conduction system.

Sinus Tachycardia—Basic Arrhythmia

Although impulse formation is normal, the rate is faster than normal in **sinus tachycardia** (Figure 4-2). Heart rate is from 100 to 160 beats per minute. P wave formation is normal but occurs closer to the preceding T wave. Other ECG characteristics are similar to normal sinus rhythm.

Clinical application: Sinus tachycardia (ST) is a normal reaction to physiological stress. However, if the heart rate is so fast that cardiac output is decreased, there is an increased oxygen demand by the myocardium. Causes of ST include exercise, fever, anxiety, and hypovolemia (decreased body fluid volume).

■ ***sinus tachycardia (ST):*** *impulse originates in SA node with a heart rate of 100 to 160 beats per minute*

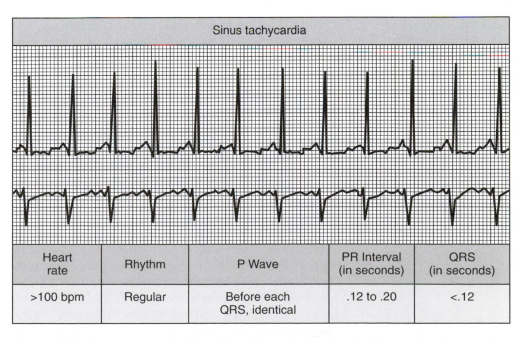

Heart rate	Rhythm	P Wave	PR Interval (in seconds)	QRS (in seconds)
>100 bpm	Regular	Before each QRS, identical	.12 to .20	<.12

Figure 4-2   Sinus tachycardia. (Copyright Marquette Electronics, Marquette, Wisconsin)

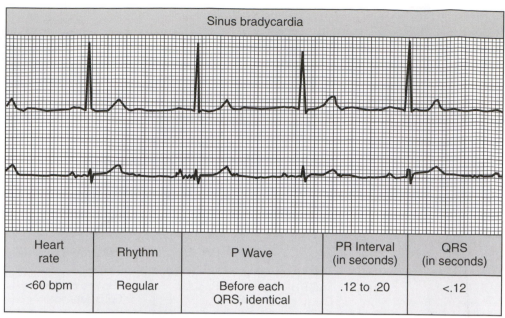

| | Sinus bradycardia | | | |

Heart rate	Rhythm	P Wave	PR Interval (in seconds)	QRS (in seconds)
<60 bpm	Regular	Before each QRS, identical	.12 to .20	<.12

Figure 4-3   Sinus bradycardia. (Copyright Marquette Electronics, Marquette, Wisconsin)

Sinus Bradycardia—Basic Arrhythmia

The rate is slower than normal in **sinus bradycardia,** although impulse formation occurs normally (Figure 4-3). Heart rate is between 30 and 60 beats per minute. If the heart rate is too slow, cardiac output is decreased.

Clinical application: Symptoms of decreased cardiac output include angina, palpitations, syncope (fainting), dizziness, hypotension, shortness of breath, and decreased peripheral perfusion (blood flow). Bradycardia may occur during vomiting, suctioning of the trachea, a valsalva maneuver, or from certain drug effects. Healthy, conditioned athletes may also possess lower than normal heart rates.

Sinus Arrhythmia—Basic Arrhythmia

During **sinus arrhythmia,** impulses originate from the SA node, but speed up with inspiration of air and slow down with expiration of air. ECG characteristics are similar to normal sinus rhythm except the P-P and R-R intervals vary slightly (Figure 4-4).

Sinus Arrest or Pause—Possible Lethal Basic Arrhythmia

When the SA node fails momentarily to initiate an impulse, **sinus arrest** occurs (Figure 4-5); **sinus pause** happens when the impulses are prevented from leaving the SA node (Figure 4-6). There is no atrial activity without stimulation of the atria to contract. Long pauses in which beats are dropped appear on the ECG. In sinus arrest, a complete P, QRS, or T cycle is missing and results in a sudden decrease in cardiac output. The ECG characteristics appear normal in the beats that do occur, but are absent in the arrest or pause beats. Heart rate may be variable and the rhythm is irregular due to skipped beats. Sinus arrest occurs if there is a prolonged failure of SA node automaticity longer than three seconds. If sinus arrest or pause is transient, the consequences may be insignificant. Serious dysrhythmia is present when the episodes become repetitive or prolonged. This sudden decrease in cardiac output can cause dizziness, syncope, fatigue, or angina. An alternative or secondary pacemaker may assume and maintain the heartbeat in the case of severely delayed or even permanent

■ *sinus bradycardia:* impulse originates in SA node with a heart rate of 30 to 60 beats per minute

■ *sinus arrhythmia:* normal impulse formation that varies with respiration

Hint: *Sinus arrhythmia may occur normally in children and young adults.*

■ *sinus arrest: failure of the SA node to initiate an impulse*

■ *sinus pause: condition in which impulses are prevented from leaving the SA node*

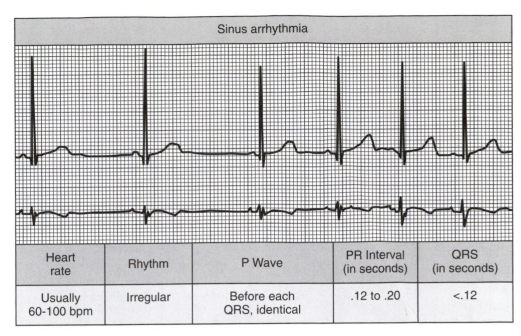

Heart rate	Rhythm	P Wave	PR Interval (in seconds)	QRS (in seconds)
Usually 60-100 bpm	Irregular	Before each QRS, identical	.12 to .20	<.12

Figure 4-4   Sinus arrhythmia. (Copyright Marquette Electronics, Marquette, Wisconsin)

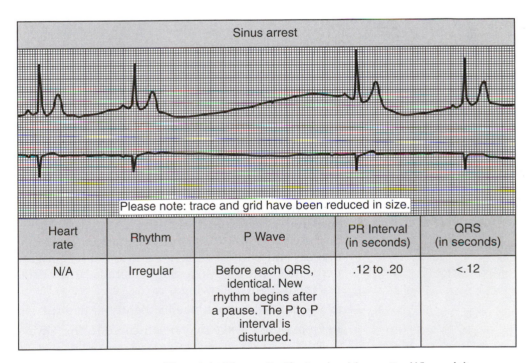

Please note: trace and grid have been reduced in size.

Heart rate	Rhythm	P Wave	PR Interval (in seconds)	QRS (in seconds)
N/A	Irregular	Before each QRS, identical. New rhythm begins after a pause. The P to P interval is disturbed.	.12 to .20	<.12

Figure 4-5   Sinus arrest. (Copyright Marquette Electronics, Marquette, Wisconsin)

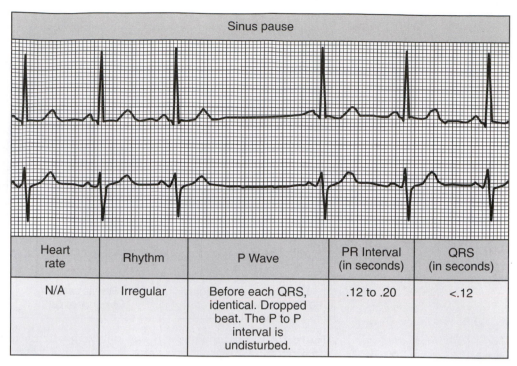

Heart rate	Rhythm	P Wave	PR Interval (in seconds)	QRS (in seconds)
N/A	Irregular	Before each QRS, identical. Dropped beat. The P to P interval is undisturbed.	.12 to .20	<.12

Figure 4-6 Sinus pause. (Copyright Marquette Electronics, Marquette, Wisconsin)

SA node cessation. A permanent pacemaker may be needed when the SA node is unable to restore normal pacing.

■ ATRIAL ARRHYTHMIAS

■ *atrial arrhythmia: abnormal electrical activity originating in the atria*

An **atrial arrhythmia** is abnormal electrical activity occurring in the atria before a normal sinus impulse can occur.

Premature Atrial Contractions—Advanced Arrhythmia

■ *premature atrial contraction (PAC): early, isolated firing of an ectopic or abnormal atrial focus*

Premature beats are the result of an isolated early atrial firing from an ectopic focus in the atria, creating waves that appear earlier than usual in the cycle. **Premature atrial contractions (PACs)** produce an early abnormal P wave because the impulse does not originate in the SA node. Because the AV node recognizes and transmits the impulse as if it had originated in the SA node, the PAC depolarizes the atria in a manner similar to a normal impulse. ECG characteristics include the following:

- Shorter P-P interval due to slightly different P wave morphology
- Premature P wave may be obscured in the T wave or QRS complex
- Abnormal P wave configuration (flat, notched, slurred, inverted, wide, or diphasic)
- R-R interval is shorter than normal
- P-R interval may be longer or shorter, depending on site of ectopic focus in the atrium
- QRS is usually normal

(See Figures 4-7, 4-8, and 4-9.)

Clinical application: PACs may result from use of alcohol, caffeine, or nicotine; low serum potassium levels; or heart or lung disease.

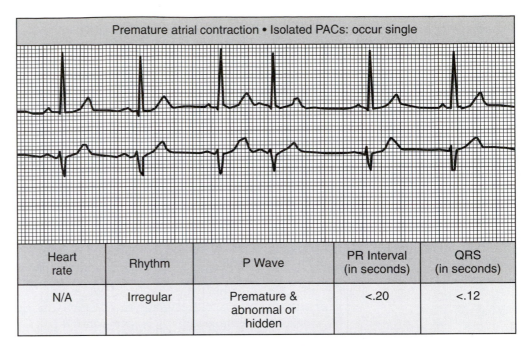

Heart rate	Rhythm	P Wave	PR Interval (in seconds)	QRS (in seconds)
N/A	Irregular	Premature & abnormal or hidden	<.20	<.12

Figure 4-7   Premature atrial contraction (PAC)—isolated. (Copyright Marquette Electronics, Marquette, Wisconsin)

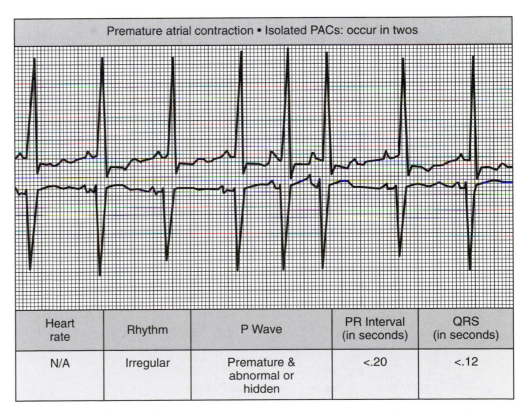

Heart rate	Rhythm	P Wave	PR Interval (in seconds)	QRS (in seconds)
N/A	Irregular	Premature & abnormal or hidden	<.20	<.12

Figure 4-8   PAC—paired. (Copyright Marquette Electronics, Marquette, Wisconsin)

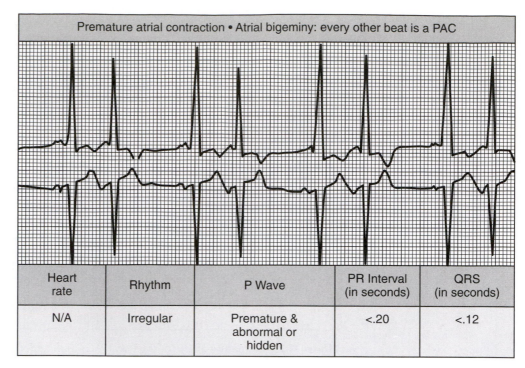

	Premature atrial contraction • Atrial bigeminy: every other beat is a PAC			
Heart rate	Rhythm	P Wave	PR Interval (in seconds)	QRS (in seconds)
N/A	Irregular	Premature & abnormal or hidden	<.20	<.12

Figure 4-9 PAC—bigeminy. (Copyright Marquette Electronics, Marquette, Wisconsin)

Atrial Tachycardias—Advanced Arrhythmia

■ *supraventricular tachycardia (SVT):* an atrial ectopic focus with a heart rate of 150 to 200 beats per minute

Atrial tachycardia or **supraventricular tachycardia (SVT)** occurs with a sudden onset of an ectopic atrial focus. The P wave configuration differs from sinus P waves and is difficult to see, as it may be superimposed on the preceding T wave (Figure 4-10). The atrial heart rate is 150 to 200 beats per minute, while the ventricular rate varies with the degree of block. If there is no block, the ventricular rate is the same as the atrial rate. The rhythm is regular with abnormal conduction in the ventricles. With atrial tachycardia there is decreased cardiac output due to the fast heart rate and an increased oxygen demand by the myocardium.

Atrial Fibrillation—Possible Lethal Basic Arrhythmia

■ *atrial fibrillation:* multiple ectopic foci discharging impulses very rapidly

Atrial fibrillation occurs when multiple ectopic foci in the atria discharge impulses at a very rapid rate and override the SA node. Although firing very rapidly, each impulse, or atrial fibrillation, results in depolarization of only a small portion of the atrial myocardium rather than the whole atrium. Without uniform atrial depolarization, there is no P wave. This chaotic firing produces an ECG deflection known as an "f" wave. These waves vary in size and shape and are irregular in rhythm (Figure 4-11). ECG characteristics include:

■ No true P waves; "f" waves instead

■ QRS complex is normal

■ Indeterminate P-R interval

■ Rate and rhythm: atrial is irregular and 400 to 600 beats per minute; ventricular is irregular and varies with the degree of AV block

Clinical application: Atrial fibrillation is usually the result of underlying heart disease. It may occur intermittently or as a chronic rhythm. Clot formation from stagnation of blood in the atria may cause thrombus on the wall of the heart, predisposing the patient to pulmonary embolism or cerebral vascular accident.

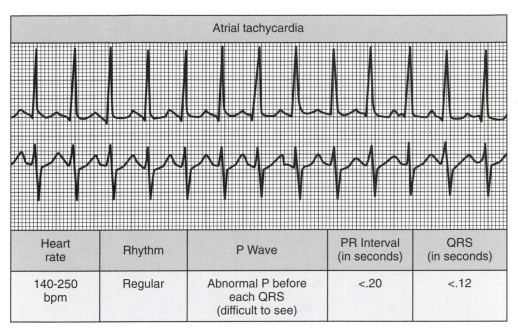

Heart rate	Rhythm	P Wave	PR Interval (in seconds)	QRS (in seconds)
140-250 bpm	Regular	Abnormal P before each QRS (difficult to see)	<.20	<.12

Figure 4-10   Atrial tachycardia. (Copyright Marquette Electronics, Marquette, Wisconsin)

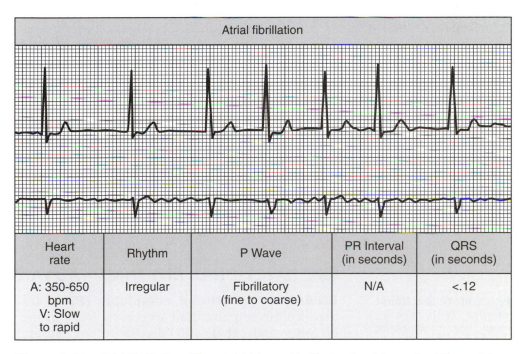

Heart rate	Rhythm	P Wave	PR Interval (in seconds)	QRS (in seconds)
A: 350-650 bpm V: Slow to rapid	Irregular	Fibrillatory (fine to coarse)	N/A	<.12

Figure 4-11   Atrial fibrillation. (Copyright Marquette Electronics, Marquette, Wisconsin)

Atrial Flutter—Advanced Arrhythmia

■ *atrial flutter: a sawtooth pattern resulting from an ectopic atrial focus*

In **atrial flutter,** an ectopic atrial focus generates impulses faster than the SA node and takes over the function of cardiac pacemaker. Each P wave appears identical to all the others, because they are discharged from the same ectopic focus. The P waves resemble a sawtooth pattern or picket fence appearance (Figure 4-12). A protective mechanism within the AV node prevents a certain ratio of the stimuli from reaching the ventricles. Rapid ventricular rates pose a threat to the patient. For example, if the atrial rate (or number of P waves) is 300 per minute and the AV node blocks every third P wave, then the ventricular rate is

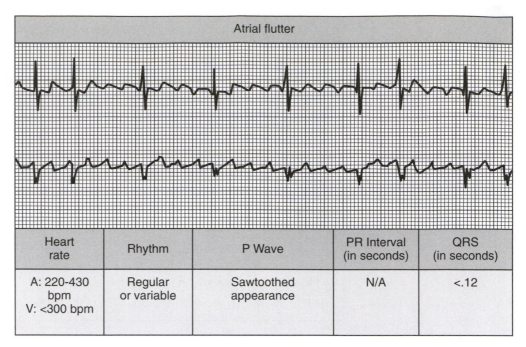

Heart rate	Rhythm	P Wave	PR Interval (in seconds)	QRS (in seconds)
A: 220-430 bpm V: <300 bpm	Regular or variable	Sawtoothed appearance	N/A	<.12

Figure 4-12 Atrial flutter. (Copyright Marquette Electronics, Marquette, Wisconsin)

100 per minute. This tracing on the ECG is described as atrial flutter with a 2:1 block (2 P waves for every QRS). ECG characteristics include:

■ P waves resembling a sawtooth pattern
■ P-R interval is not measurable
■ QRS complex is normal
■ atrial rate is 250 to 350 per minute; ventricular rate varies with the degree of AV block
■ atrial rhythm is regular and ventricular rhythm is usually regular

Clinical application: Atrial flutter may occur in pulmonary disease and congestive heart failure.

▬▬▬ JUNCTIONAL RHYTHMS—ADVANCED ARRHYTHMIA

■ *premature junctional complex (PJC): an early impulse from an ectopic focus near the AV node*

Premature junctional complexes (PJCs) are impulses transpiring earlier than a sinus impulse from an ectopic focus in the region of the AV node. The PJC allows retrograde atrial depolarization, causing the P wave to become negative or inverted. ECG characteristics are as follows:

■ P waves are negative and may occur before, during, or after the QRS complex.
■ P-R interval may be shortened or not measurable.
■ QRS is usually normal.
■ Rate is determined by sinus rhythm and the number of PJCs.
■ Rhythm is irregular due to premature beats.
■ Conduction: atrial is retrograde; ventricular is usually normal.

Premature junctional complexes may predispose the heart to more serious dysrhythmias (Figures 4-13 and 4-14).

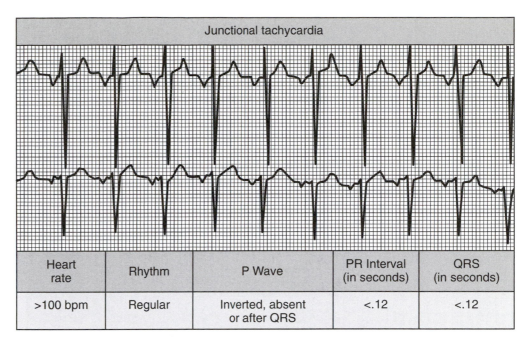

Heart rate	Rhythm	P Wave	PR Interval (in seconds)	QRS (in seconds)
>100 bpm	Regular	Inverted, absent or after QRS	<.12	<.12

Figure 4-13 Junctional rhythms. (Copyright Marquette Electronics, Marquette, Wisconsin)

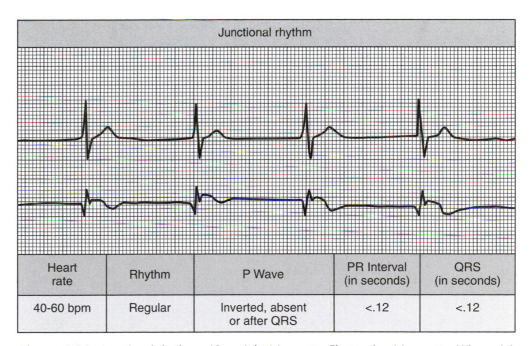

Heart rate	Rhythm	P Wave	PR Interval (in seconds)	QRS (in seconds)
40-60 bpm	Regular	Inverted, absent or after QRS	<.12	<.12

Figure 4-14 Junctional rhythms. (Copyright Marquette Electronics, Marquette, Wisconsin)

▨▨▨ VENTRICULAR RHYTHMS

In a ventricular rhythm, an ectopic focus in the bundle branches, Purkinje fibers, or ventricular muscle initiates an impulse before the impulse from the underlying rhythm can be generated.

Premature Ventricular Contractions—Advanced Arrhythmia

■ *premature ventricular contraction (PVC): an early impulse beginning in either ventricle*

In a **premature ventricular contraction (PVC),** the ectopic focus, a depolarization originating in either ventricle prematurely, stimulates the ventricle to

■ **couplets:** *two PVCs*

■ **salvo:** *three or more sequential PVCs*

■ **ventricular bigeminy:** *a heart rhythm in which every other beat is a PVC*

■ **ventricular trigeminy:** *a heart rhythm in which every third beat is a PVC*

■ **ventricular quadrigeminy:** *a heart rhythm in which every fourth beat is a PVC*

contract before the next sinus beat can be conducted to the ventricles. Because the normal sequence of ventricular depolarization is altered, the ventricles depolarize sequentially rather than simultaneously. Impulse conduction happens through the myocardium instead of over the normal conduction pathways. This aberrant path causes a wide and frequently bizarre-appearing QRS. PVCs exist in multiple types of configurations (Figures 4-15, 4-16, and 4-17). Two PVCs together are **couplets** or pairs. A **salvo** consists of three or more sequential PVCs. **Ventricular bigeminy** arises when every other beat is a PVC; **ventricular trigeminy** is every third beat; **ventricular quadrigeminy** is every fourth beat. The ECG characteristics of a PVC are as follows:

■ P wave is usually absent.

■ P-R interval is nonexistent.

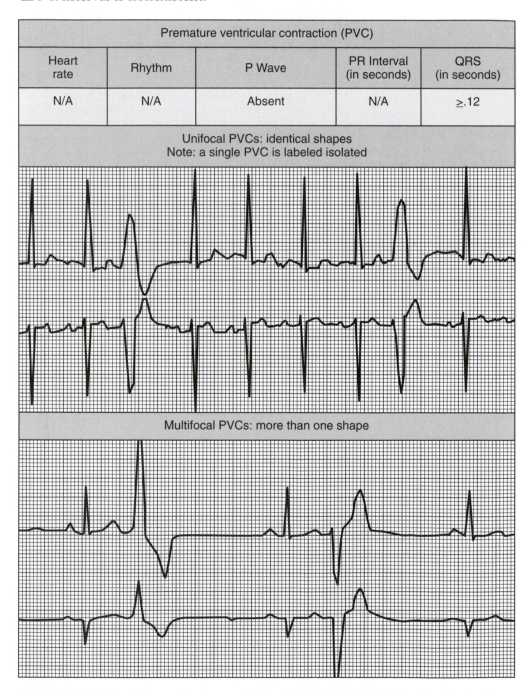

Premature ventricular contraction (PVC)				
Heart rate	Rhythm	P Wave	PR Interval (in seconds)	QRS (in seconds)
N/A	N/A	Absent	N/A	≥.12

Figure 4-15 Premature ventricular contraction (PVC). (Copyright Marquette Electronics, Marquette, Wisconsin)

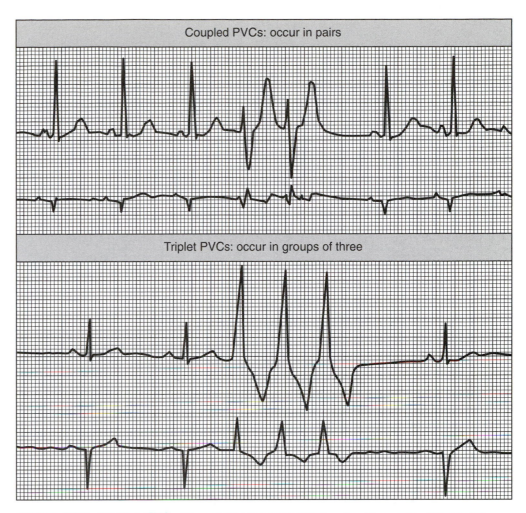

Figure 4-16   Multiple PVCs. (Copyright Marquette Electronics, Marquette, Wisconsin)

- QRS complex is premature, bizarre, widened, and notched. The complex may be of greater amplitude than a sinus QRS complex.
- Rate is determined by the underlying rate and number of PVCs.
- Rhythm: atrial is irregular, due to retrograde conduction of the PVC; ventricular is irregular because of the premature beats.
- Conduction is abnormal.

Clinical application: PVCs reduce cardiac output because of the decreased time for the ventricles to fill with blood in diastole. Gastric overload, stress, electrolyte imbalance, and excessive use of alcohol, nicotine, and caffeine may manifest on the ECG as PVCs.

Ventricular Tachycardia—Possible Lethal Basic Arrhythmia

■ ventricular tachycardia (VT): *ventricular ectopic discharge at a rapid, regular rate in excess of 100 beats per minute*

If three or more impulses of ventricular ectopic origin discharge in a succession of rapid, regular impulses at rates in excess of 100 per minute, **ventricular tachycardia (VT)** is present (Figure 4-18). In association with myocardial infarction, VT may represent a life-threatening situation. ECG characteristics present as:

- P waves are nonexistent.
- P-R interval is absent.
- QRS complexes are consecutive, wide, and bizarre.
- Rate is 100 to 250 per minute.

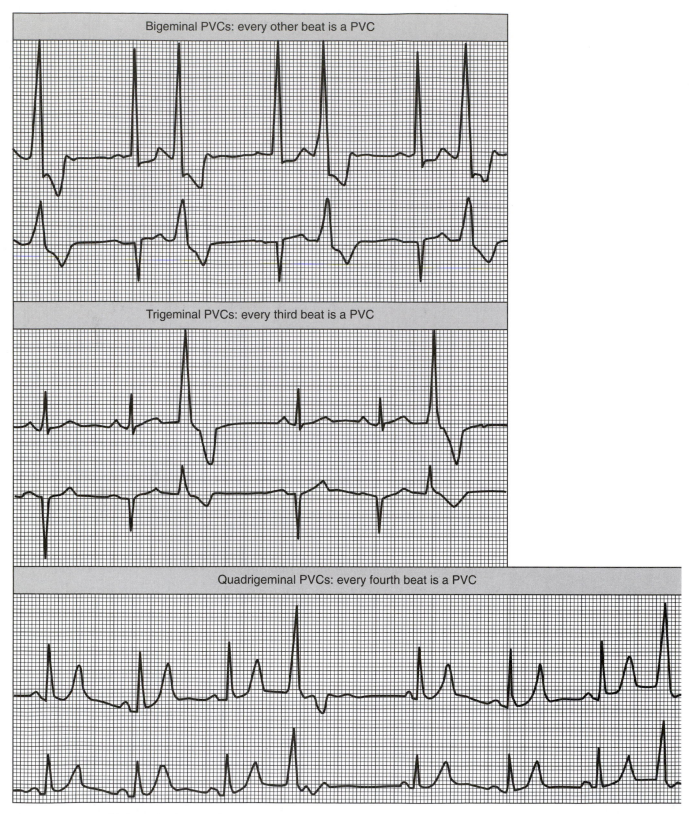

Figure 4-17   Multiple PVCs. (Copyright Marquette Electronics, Marquette, Wisconsin)

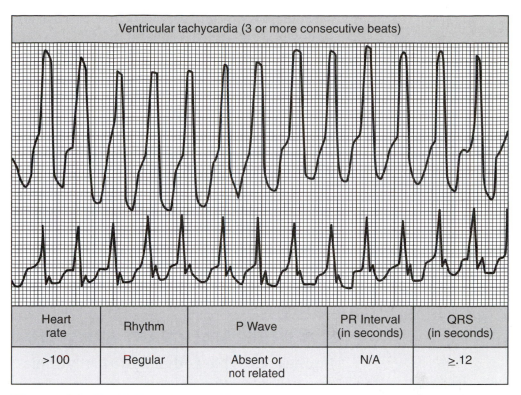

Heart rate	Rhythm	P Wave	PR Interval (in seconds)	QRS (in seconds)
>100	Regular	Absent or not related	N/A	≥.12

Figure 4-18   Ventricular tachycardia. (Copyright Marquette Electronics, Marquette, Wisconsin)

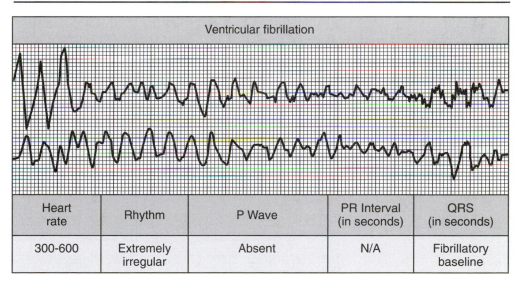

Heart rate	Rhythm	P Wave	PR Interval (in seconds)	QRS (in seconds)
300-600	Extremely irregular	Absent	N/A	Fibrillatory baseline

Figure 4-19   Ventricular fibrillation. (Copyright Marquette Electronics, Marquette, Wisconsin)

- Rhythm is generally regular.
- Conduction is abnormal.

Ventricular tachycardia reflects decreased or no cardiac output deteriorating into ventricular fibrillation.

Ventricular Fibrillation—Possible Lethal Basic Arrhythmia

■ **ventricular fibrillation (VF):** *chaotic, ventricular rhythm as a result of multiple foci*

Ventricular fibrillation (VF) exists when the ventricular rhythm is chaotic, resulting from multiple areas within the ventricle exhibiting varying degrees of depolarization and repolarization. This rapid discharge of impulses results in quivering, not contracting, of the ventricles; therefore, there is no cardiac output or blood in the coronary arteries (Figure 4-19). VF is created by the attempt of multiple ventricular sites to assume pacemaking by firing simultaneously in an attempt to increase cardiac output. The ECG appearance is as follows:

- P waves are absent.
- P-R interval is nonexistent.
- QRS complexes are not present.
- No rate or rhythm exists.
- Conduction is abnormal.

Clinical application: Basic life support measures must be instituted immediately in an attempt to maintain the life of the patient.

ATRIOVENTRICULAR BLOCK—ADVANCED ARRHYTHMIA

■ **atrioventricular block (AV block):** *condition in which the conduction system delays or blocks an electrical impulse at any given point in the conduction system*

In **atrioventricular block (AV),** the conduction system delays or blocks the electrical transmission at some point in the pathway. The most common blocks arise at the AV node, the bundle of His, or the bundle branches. This abnormal or delayed disturbance may be transient or permanent.

OTHER MALIGNANT ARRHYTHMIAS

Agonal—Possible Lethal Basic Arrhythmia

■ **agonal rhythm:** *irregular and widely spaced complexes originating from ventricular ectopic foci*

An **agonal rhythm** consists of very irregular and widely spaced complexes originating from several different ventricular pacemakers. Agonal rhythm has a very poor prognosis.

Asystole—Possible Lethal Basic Arrhythmia

■ **asystole:** *absence of heart contraction*

Because no ventricular depolarization occurs in **asystole,** there is no contraction of the heart. Because there is no mechanical or electrical cardiac activity, asystole shows up as an isoelectric line on the ECG (Figure 4-20). With an extremely poor prognosis, asystole may be the final result of other malignant rhythms, the initial event in cardiac arrest, or the result of ventricular fibrillation.

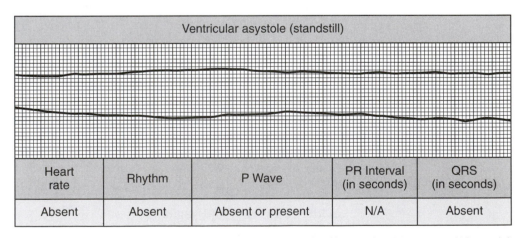

Heart rate	Rhythm	P Wave	PR Interval (in seconds)	QRS (in seconds)
Absent	Absent	Absent or present	N/A	Absent

Figure 4-20   Ventricular asystole. (Copyright Marquette Electronics, Marquette, Wisconsin)

REVIEW QUESTIONS

Multiple Choice Questions

1. In sinus rhythm, the heartbeat originates in the:
   a. AV node.
   b. sinus node.
   c. AV junction.
   d. SA node.

2. The normal heart rate established by the SA node is:
   a. 40 to 60 beats per minute.
   b. 75 beats per minute.
   c. 20 to 40 beats per minute.
   d. 60 to 100 beats per minute.

3. Dysrhythmia refers to:
   a. an abnormality in rhythm.
   b. an absence of rhythm.
   c. a combination of abnormality and absence of rhythm.

4. Sinus tachycardia represents:
   a. an increase in the rate of discharge of the sinus node.
   b. a decrease in the rate of discharge of the sinus node.
   c. an increase in the rate of discharge of the atrioventricular node.
   d. a decrease in the rate of discharge of the atrioventricular node.

5. Premature atrial stimulation from an atrial ectopic focus produces an early abnormal _____ wave.
   a. R
   b. QRS
   c. T
   d. P

Matching Questions

Match each term with the letter of the correct definition.

6. dysrhythmia
7. atrial fibrillation
8. sinus arrest
9. sinus tachycardia
10. PAC
11. atrial flutter
12. asystole
13. sinus arrhythmia
14. ectopic
15. agonal arrhythmia
    a. early, isolated firing of an ectopic atrial focus
    b. abnormality in heart rhythm
    c. a sawtooth pattern resulting from an ectopic atrial focus
    d. sinus impulse, heart rate 100 to 160 beats per minute
    e. multiple ectopic foci discharging impulses at a very rapid rate
    f. normal impulse formation that varies with respiration
    g. absence of heart contraction
    h. failure of SA node to initiate an impulse
    i. a conduction impulse formed in an aberrant site
    j. irregular and widely spaced complexes originating from ventricular ectopic foci

Short Answer/Fill in the Blank

16. Ventricular asystole represents the total _____ of ventricular activity.

17. A _____ is two PVCs.

18. Ventricular _____ is chaotic ventricular rhythm as a result of multiple foci.

19. Atrial tachycardia or SVT occurs with the sudden onset of an ectopic _____ focus.

CHAPTER 5

Acquiring the ECG

OBJECTIVES:

After reading this chapter, you will be able to:

Demonstrate correct use of ECG equipment.

Perform simple maintenance and troubleshoot ECG equipment.

Perform accurate, diagnostic ECGs for physician interpretation in numerous situations and circumstances.

Understand the importance of patient preparation for testing procedures.

Explain the effects of patient position.

Understand the concept of electrical conduction through the skin.

Demonstrate proper skin preparation and lead placement.

Recognize artifact on ECG and practice good artifact prevention.

OVERVIEW

Performance of a diagnostic ECG depends on a well-trained technician and reliable equipment. It is equally important to maintain the equipment. It is essential to remember that the ECG you are performing is a diagnostic test. The physician will be making treatment decisions based upon the tracings obtained on the ECG. This chapter examines numerous procedural considerations that must be taken into account to ensure that the ECG is accurate and of the best diagnostic quality possible to provide information on cardiac status. The interpretation, diagnosis, and treatment depend on the accuracy of the ECG tracings. This chapter discusses the importance of patient preparation and positioning, skin preparation, and recognition of artifact in proper ECG recordings.

Certain patient pathology and extrinsic situations may alter the choice of site from standard electrode placement. In these cases, position the electrode as close as possible to the correct site and document the change on the ECG. It is essential to inform the interpreting physician of special circumstances by documentation on the ECG.

EQUIPMENT OPERATION

Newer ECG analysis systems are battery powered and can record, display, print, store, and transmit multiple channels of ECG data simultaneously. This kind of electrocardiograph is known as a *multichannel system*. Some models will record a 15-lead pediatric ECG as well as the conventional 12-lead adult ECG. The automatic, multichannel system switches leads internally (Figure 5-1). A manual, 12-lead, single-channel ECG (which may still be used at some facilities) records only one lead at a time (Figures 5-2 and 5-3). A multichannel instrument saves time and paper as compared to the single-channel model. ECG instruments may be placed on portable carts, making the ECG one of the most portable diagnostic tests available (Figure 5-4).

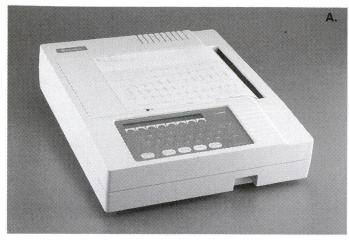

A.

Figure 5-1   A. Multichannel ECG machine (Courtesy of Siemens Burdick, Inc.) B. 3-channel ECG recording

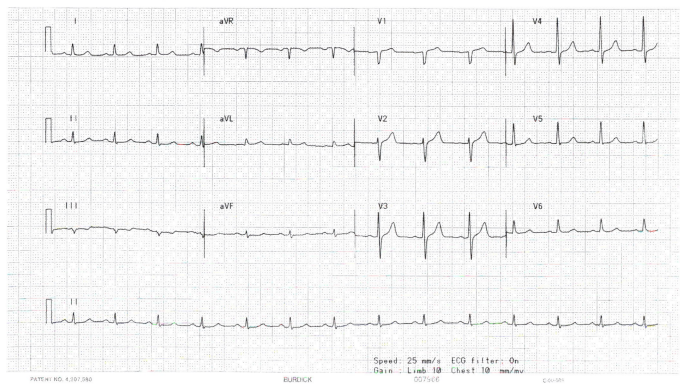

Speed: 25 mm/s   ECG filter: On
Gain : Limb 10 Chest 10 mm/mv

PATENT NO. 4,207,580   BURDICK   007966   C-00-501

B.

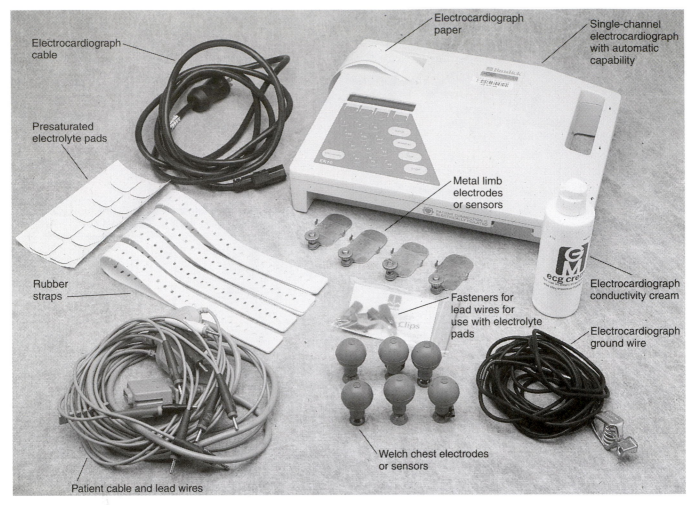

Figure 5-2   Single-channel ECG

Advanced systems can transmit ECG data via telephone line to a central receiving device for printout and interpretation. Interpretation may be completed by a physician or a computer or a combination of the two. The completed, interpreted ECG may be faxed to other facilities. Systems with storage capabilities can even transmit portions of previous ECGs of the patient, if desired for comparison.

A standard 12-lead ECG instrument is composed of 10 lead wires connected to sensing electrodes on the surface of the patient's skin. (Two electrodes are switched automatically and used twice.) Electrical activity of the heart is detected by the sensing electrodes and transmitted by the lead wires, which connect to the galvanometer of the instrument. The electrical signals are magnified by the amplifier, changed into motion from voltage, and recorded on the recording paper by the stylus.

MAINTENANCE OF EQUIPMENT

Cleaning and Care of Equipment

Most ECG carts may be cleaned with a soft cloth and a mild detergent diluted with water. Make sure that the ECG cart AC power "on/off" switch is in the "off" position and that the cart is unplugged from the electrical outlet. Wring the cloth until damp and wipe the exterior of the system. Do not wipe the open vents, connectors, plugs, or the writer. The acquisition module may also be cleaned in this manner, but avoid contact with the lead wire connectors.

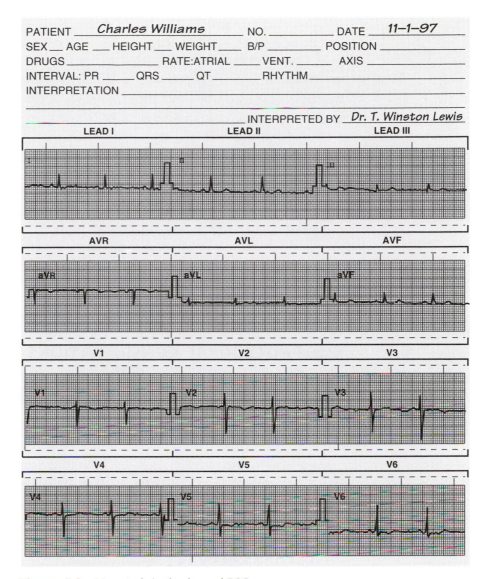

PATIENT ___*Charles Williams*___ NO. _____ DATE ___*11–1–97*___
SEX __ AGE ___ HEIGHT ___ WEIGHT ___ B/P _____ POSITION _____
DRUGS _____ RATE:ATRIAL ___ VENT. _____ AXIS _____
INTERVAL: PR _____ QRS _____ QT _____ RHYTHM _____
INTERPRETATION _____
_____
_____ INTERPRETED BY ___*Dr. T. Winston Lewis*___

Figure 5-3 Mounted single-channel ECG

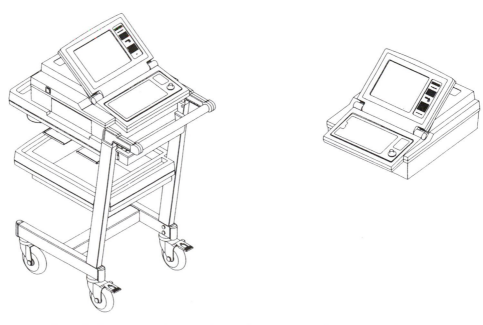

Figure 5-4 ECG system with cart. (Copyright Marquette Electronics, Marquette, Wisconsin)

Clinical application:

■ The lead wires should always be placed over the handle or over the top of the cart, never tied or bent.

■ The cart should be wiped with a damp cloth at once a day.

■ Inspect the lead wires and clips for breaks or cracks.

■ Never put foods or liquids on carts. The carts have computer keyboards that will be damaged by spillage.

■ Inspect the wheels for anything that may become caught, making the cart difficult to steer.

■ Never write or place anything on the ECG monitor screen. It will break.

■ Always plug the cart into a wall electrical outlet when not in use. Many carts are battery-powered. The battery cannot recharge if it is not plugged into an outlet.

■ Inspect electrical cords for fraying or other damage; inspect plugs and connectors for bent prongs or pins. Enlist qualified service personnel to repair or replace.

■ Follow any recommendations of the equipment manufacturer.

PROCEDURAL CONSIDERATIONS

Patient Preparation

When an ECG is ordered by a physician, make sure that you have the proper patient. If the patient is conscious, ask him to state his name; if the patient is unconscious, check his wristband; in trauma situations, perform the ECG and verify identity later.

As a health care provider, it is essential that you maintain personal hygiene and dress and speak professionally. An impression of competence will inspire patient confidence in the health care provider. Introduce yourself; smile and explain your role in the care of the patient. Maintain eye contact with the patient. Using the patient's name in any conversation indicates respect and consideration for the individual. Explain the ECG procedure and what the patient can expect. Emphasize that no pain is involved. This helps to reduce patient anxiety.

The patient must be as calm and quiet as possible. Promote a peaceful environment. Provide privacy. If the ECG is performed in a hospital situation, ask visitors to please leave the room until after the test. Pull the curtain and shut the door. Explain to the patient that his or her chest will be exposed during the testing process. Respect the patient's modesty. Expose only the chest and the extremities for the procedure. If the patient is cold, position the electrodes and then cover the patient with a blanket during the test.

Patient Position

A patient should always be placed in a supine position when an ECG is being done. Lying on either side or elevation of the chest may alter the position of the heart within the chest. Criteria for normal ECGs are based on patients in the supine position. Because the vectors are affected by body position, the physician interpreting the test requires all pertinent information to effectively and correctly evaluate the cardiac status. If the patient cannot lie flat, lower the patient to the lowest comfortable position and document the approximate angle between the patient and the examination table or bed.

Clinical application: Head of bed (HOB) is 45 degrees for a patient who is short of breath; HOB is 30 degrees for a patient with a head injury.

Skin Preparation

Accurate ECG tracings depend on optimal contact between skin and the electrode. Poor electrode adherence to the skin interface is a common source of

■ **epidermis:** *the outermost layer of skin cells*

■ **dermis:** *the middle skin layer just under the epidermis*

problems that contribute to a nondiagnostic ECG. The skin is composed of three layers, each with different electrical conductivity. The upper skin layer, the **epidermis,** consists of dead skin cells, which are very resistant and provide poor electrical conduction. A less resistant and better conducting layer, the **dermis,** lies beneath the epidermis. The dermis is composed of living cells and is the layer of skin needed to detect electrical signals for the ECG.

For adequate electrode contact, dead skin, hair, oil, and any other deterrent or resistance to conductivity must be removed. Providing an electrode-to-skin interface is crucial for detection of electrical signals from the heart. The following skin preparation techniques should be used on all individuals:

■ Shave any chest hair, where appropriate, from each electrode site. Carefully dry-shave chest with a disposable razor, using short strokes in one direction. Dispose of razor using standard precautions. Shaving improves conductivity, holds the electrode to the skin, and allows easy removal of the electrode upon test completion. Stock razors on the ECG cart for excess hair removal.

■ Use an alcohol wipe to remove excess oil from the skin. Allow the wiped spot to air-dry.

■ Thoroughly abrade each electrode site with a 4 × 4 gauze pad or a special ultrafine sandpaper for skin to remove loose epidermal skin cells.

■ Finally, apply electrodes in correct chest and limb placement. Some electrodes incorporate a conductive wet gel in the center, surrounded by an adhesive pad. Other electrodes are dry gel tabs that leave no residue upon removal (Figure 5-5). Apply upper extremity and chest electrode tabs so that the tabs are in a downward position; apply lower extremity tabs so that the tabs are in an upward position. These tab positions permit improved connection with the lead wires by lessening tension on the lead wires.

Clinical application: If a patient is **diaphoretic,** try to remove perspiration with a 4 × 4 gauze pad and swab with alcohol if necessary.

■ **diaphoretic:** *producing perspiration; sweating*

Clinical application: Apply pressure for adhesion at the electrode edge, not in the center, so gel will not dislodge from electrode. ▦ **Rationale:** *A good ECG recording depends on current flowing between the dermis through the conductive gel of the electrode.* ▦

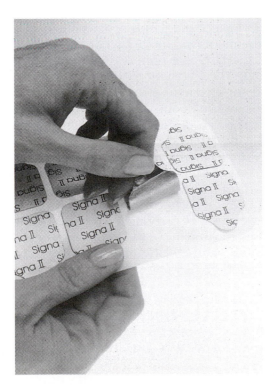

Figure 5-5 Disposable electrodes. (Courtesy of Siemens Burdick, Inc.)

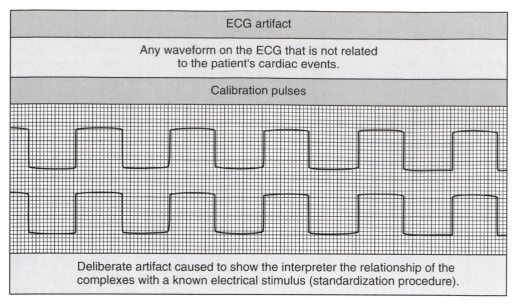

| ECG artifact |
| Any waveform on the ECG that is not related to the patient's cardiac events. |
| Calibration pulses |

Deliberate artifact caused to show the interpreter the relationship of the complexes with a known electrical stimulus (standardization procedure).

Figure 5-6   ECG artifact. (Copyright Marquette Electronics, Marquette, Wisconsin)

Recognizing Artifact

The evaluation of a normal ECG is sometimes complicated by the recording of extraneous, undesirable electrical activity from sources other than the heart. Poor electrode contact, interference by other electrical devices in the immediate vicinity, and even patient movement may produce this type of interference, known as **artifact** (Figure 5-6). Some types of artifact are readily identifiable by their shapes, such as interference from electrical appliances and fluorescent lighting. AC interference is a rapid vibration that produces spikes of similar amplitude that widen the baseline and make it fuzzy and thick. In the United States, the frequency of the spikes is 60 cycles per second (Figure 5-7).

Clinical application: AC interference may be lessened by positioning the front of the ECG cart away from the patient's bed. A power cable running parallel to the bed may create AC interference. If possible, disconnect the wall plugs of any electrical appliance near the bed. This may be difficult in a critical care setting. Do not allow the feet and hands of the patient to touch any portion of the bed other than the mattress. Muscle tremor artifact may be reduced by assuring the patient that the ECG is a noninvasive procedure to measure the amount and direction of electrical activity produced by the heart. Expose only those body areas needed for electrode placement and keep the patient warm by using a blanket and a warm room. Voluntary muscle tremor may result when the patient talks, sneezes, or moves. Involuntary somatic tremor may be produced by a patient with Parkinson's disease, hyperthyroidism, or any nervous system disorder. The wave pattern may resemble the "f" waves of atrial flutter. This artifact may be lessened by positioning limb electrodes on or near the upper arms and thighs, where the tremor is less remarkable. Place the patient's hands under his or her buttocks while recording the ECG.

The baseline of the ECG should be straight. If it is "wandering" or has "sway" (Figure 5-8), repeat to remove this problem. Try re-prepping the patient and re-running the test, as the cause may be inadequate electrode contact. In chest leads, wandering baseline may be the result of excessive respiratory movement.

Clinical application: Do not allow electrodes to dry out. ▣▣ **Rationale:** *Dryness may cause artifact and wandering baseline.* ▣▣

Any ECG that shows a significant amount of artifact should be repeated. If the artifact exists after several attempts to correct the problem, the reason and number of attempts should be documented on the ECG before physician interpreta-

■ **artifact:** *interference or noise in an ECG tracing*

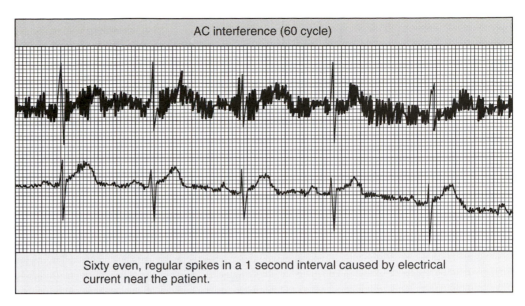

Figure 5-7 AC interference (60 cycle). (Copyright Marquette Electronics, Marquette, Wisconsin)

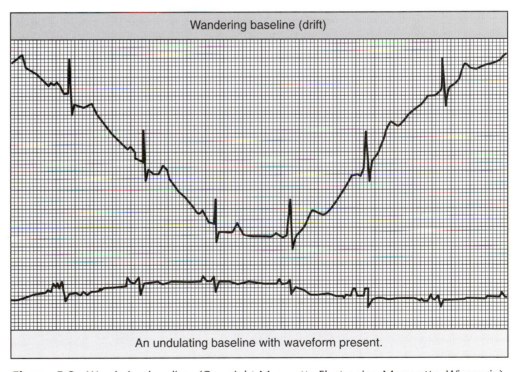

Figure 5-8 Wandering baseline. (Copyright Marquette Electronics, Marquette, Wisconsin)

tion. The physician will be unable to accurately interpret an ECG tracing with artifact. Artifact may mimic a number of dysrhythmias, especially atrial and ventricular fibrillation.

Clinical application: If you should incur artifact (tremor, 60-cycle interference, or baseline sway), the following rules will assist in determining the location and cause(s) of interference.

- If interference is in leads I and II (not III), check the right arm.
- If interference is in leads II and III (not I), check the left leg.

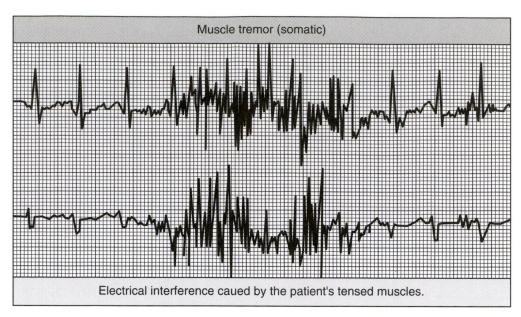

Figure 5-9   Muscle tremor. (Copyright Marquette Electronics, Marquette, Wisconsin)

- If interference is in leads I and III (not II), check the left arm.
- If interference is present in the augmented leads (AVR, AVL, and AVF), the affected limb will also display artifact (AVR—right arm; AVL—left arm; AVF—left foot).

  Additional considerations:
- Ensure that patient is lying quietly with extremities not flexed. Anxiety may cause muscle tremor artifact (Figure 5-9).
- Check for disconnected lead wires, wires not completely attached to electrode tabs, or tabs pulling away from skin.
- Place the ECG cart away from the patient's bed (if possible, at a 45-degree angle to the bed). This will prevent interference from other electrical equipment, especially in critical care units.

Errors in recording may also occur from lead reversal and lead placement errors. Suspect right and left arm lead reversal if all components of the ECG in lead I are inverted. Some ECG instruments may print "suspect lead reversal." Another cause of negative P, QRS, and T inversion is dextrocardia. The diagnosis of dextrocardia may be confirmed by comparing chest leads. Because chest leads use a unipolar lead system, they appear normal even if the limb leads are reversed. See the section on "Patient Pathology and Special Situations" later in this chapter.

Prioritization of Time for the Multiskilled Provider

As a multiskilled health care provider, you may be asked to provide more than one service at a time. It will be necessary to decide which procedure should take priority according to the needs of your patients. Working closely with your patients as a multiskilled provider, you will become familiar with their individual needs.

Clinical application: For example, if an ECG and blood tests are ordered on the same patient, it is essential to determine which is the most crucial test to perform first. ■ **Rationale:** *If patient is in a diabetic crisis, perform and process the laboratory blood test first and then proceed with the ECG. If patient is experiencing chest pain and is on the verge of a possible myocardial infarction, the ECG should be performed first, followed by the blood tests.* ■■

Upon receiving orders for multiple studies on the same patient or several patients, elicit clinical information from the ordering individual concerning priorities (STAT—at once; ASAP—as soon as possible; or routine) to enable you to make prudent decisions. It is essential to know if the patient is undergoing a preoperative or preprocedure test, because testing delays or patient abnormalities might delay completion of such procedures.

▬▬ PRACTICAL RECOMMENDATIONS IN SPECIAL CIRCUMSTANCES AND SITUATIONS

Patient Pathology and Special Situations

Clinical application:

- A congenital anomaly, known as *dextrocardia,* exists in which the left ventricle, left atrium, aortic arch, and stomach are located on the right side of the thorax. When the patient has this known rightward malposition of the heart, the right and left arm leads should be reversed and the precordial leads should be repositioned and recorded with V1 on the left, V2 on the right, and the other V leads progressing rightward to V6 (Figure 5-10). Document on ECG "right side ECG."

- Due to increased blood volume in the pregnant woman, the ECG may appear different. Do not place lower limb leads on the abdomen; put them on the upper thighs instead. Interference from the baby may occur. Document on ECG "patient is [6] months pregnant."

- ECG electrodes should never be positioned on the top of the breast, regardless of woman's breast size. If the electrodes are placed lower than normal, report that fact on the ECG. Mastectomy surgery on either side should also be recorded, because the vector of the ECG may be altered as a result of this surgery.

- If a patient has a seizure while the ECG is in progress, stay with the patient. Do not attempt to restrain the patient, only to protect him or her from injury. Call for help. Once the seizure is over, redo the test and document on ECG "s/p seizure."

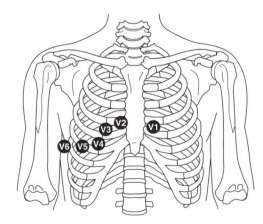

Figure 5-10   Electrode placement for dextrocardia. (Copyright Marquette Electronics, Marquette, Wisconsin)

- ECGs on limb amputees will not be affected, as all limb electrodes are positioned on the chest and abdomen.

- If a patient is contractured and unable to lie in a supine position, indicate that fact on the ECG as "contractured [right] side."

- When deviation from correct lead placement is necessary due to surgical dressings, tubes, or other extrinsic devices, include on the ECG a note such as "V2 and V3 altered due to mid-sternal dressing." Do not remove surgical dressings without a physician order. Look closely for such dressings as tegaderm. Tegaderm may adhere so tightly to the skin that it is difficult to see. If an electrode is inadvertently applied to this surface, you will be unable to obtain a tracing of the leads affected by that electrode. Never place electrodes on open wounds or burns.

- For an ECG performed during a cardiac arrest or "code" situation, or when a patient is in SVT, leave the electrodes in position if possible, as a repeat ECG may be needed. For serial recordings, the skin may also be marked with a felt marker to ensure reproducibility. Document as follows: "repeat—same lead placement." This lets the physician know that the electrodes were not removed.

- During a "trauma" or "code" situation, place the patient's name and information in the ECG cart while waiting until the ECG is needed. If there are space constraints, leave the ECG cart in the hallway whenever possible and take only the acquisition module into the room.

- For children and infants, use special pediatric electrodes for ECG testing. If unavailable or seldom required at your facility, cut standard electrodes in half lengthwise to accommodate smaller chests. Do not allow any electrode edges to touch each other (Figure 5-11).

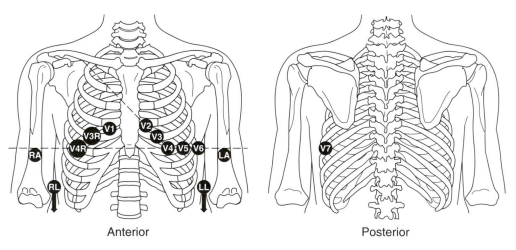

Anterior   Posterior

Place the limb (LA, LL, RA, RL) and chest (V1 through V6) leadwires, according to the standard 12-lead electrode placement.

Lead	Electrode location
V3R	Halfway between V1 and V4R.
V4R	At the mid-clavicular line in the fifth right intercostal space.
V7	At the same horizontal level of V4 in the posterior axillary line.

Figure 5-11   Pediatric electrode placement. (Copyright Marquette Electronics, Marquette, Wisconsin)

PROCEDURE

1 ECG PERFORMANCE

Equipment Required

- bed or cart for patient
- ECG cart and recording paper
- electrodes
- razors
- alcohol prep pads (70% isopropyl usually recommended)
- 4 × 4 gauze pads
- ultrafine sandpaper
- gloves, goggles, and/or impervious lab coat, if appropriate

Preparation

1. Dress, act, and speak professionally.
2. Assemble equipment needed and ECG cart.
3. Prepare the patient. Explain the procedure to reduce patient anxiety. Have patient lie in supine position.
4. Prepare the environment. Do whatever is needed to maintain privacy.

Precautions

1. Check equipment for electrical damage.
2. Check ECG cart for sufficient paper supply. If available, use different color of ECG paper for "before" physician interpretation and "after" physician interpretation.

   Note: *Green (as in first) could be provided for the "before" interpretation ECG; red (as in "read"), for the "after" physician interpretation.*

3. Wear safety equipment if appropriate. Wash hands frequently.

   Rationale: *Prevents exposure to bloodborne pathogens and spread of nosocomial infections.*

4. Wake patient if sleeping so as not to startle.
5. Have patient state full name and verify on wristband if pertinent.

   Note: *A patient may respond to someone else's name if he or she is groggy from sleep or medication. A first name is essential because patients may have similar last names. Be especially wary in trauma situations and unconscious patients.*

6. Patient must be supine.

   Rationale: *Vectors of the heart may change if patient is elevated or lying on side.*

Procedure

1. Verify the orders for the ECG.
2. Report noncompliance to nurse in charge to be properly documented and rescheduled if necessary.
3. Obtain ECG cart and equipment.
4. Greet the patient. Wake patient if sleeping.
5. Introduce yourself. Explain your role in the care of the patient.
6. Explain the ECG procedure and what to expect.
7. Provide privacy for patient.
8. Positively identify the patient. Have patient state name. Verify information on wristband for facility-based patients. Patient may be further identified by Social Security number or institutional number.
9. Place patient in supine position.
10. Prepare skin for electrodes by shaving chest hair, removing excess oil, and abrading electrode area with a 4 × 4 gauze pad.
11. Apply electrodes in correct limb and chest lead placement.

    a. The chest leads are placed using designated bony landmarks as a guide. For locating the first rib, use the clavicle as a reference point. The first intercostal space is considered to be the area between the first and second ribs. V1 is located in the fourth intercostal space to the right of the sternum. To find the fourth intercostal space, count the ribs. Find the clavicle on the right side. The clavicle is considered the first rib. Using your right hand, place your forefinger in the space below the clavicle. This is the first intercostal space. Find the next rib with your middle finger. The space below that rib is the second intercostal space. Leave your middle finger there. Using your next finger, find the third intercostal space. With your little finger, find the fourth intercostal

continues

space and place the first electrode, V1, there. Place V2 directly across from V1 at the left sternal border. V4 is positioned at the midclavicular line in the fifth intercostal space. V3 is then positioned halfway between leads V2 and V4. V5 and V6 are located laterally to V4. V5 is in the anterior axillary line and V6 is in the midaxillary line. In females, leads V4 and V5 are situated on the chest wall beneath the breast. Placing electrodes on bony protuberances will cause artifact from interference (Figure 5-12).

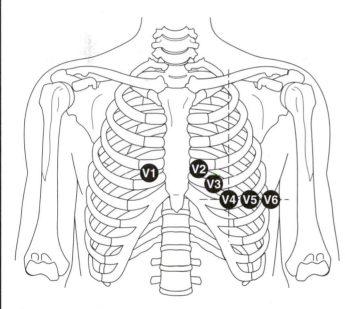

Figure 5-12 Electrode placement

   b. Place electrodes on patient first and then enter information into ECG cart.

     Rationale: *This allows the electrode gel to make contact with the skin.*

12. Attach correct lead wire on acquisition module to appropriate electrode. Lead wires are color-coded and labeled for easier attachment.

Clinical application: Right and left lead reversal should be suspected when all the components (P, QRS, and T) in lead I of the ECG are inverted (negative). Dextrocardia will also cause negative deflections in lead I. Suspect right arm and left leg reversal when the P wave is negative in leads I, II, and III. The chest leads are a unipolar system and do

not reflect lead reversal; that is, they will appear normal even if the limb leads are reversed. Repeat if necessary. Some ECG carts will show "limb lead reversal" on the screen.

     Note: *Verify correct lead placement after the leads are positioned, before recording the ECG, and as you remove the electrode patches afterwards. A physician will also notice limb lead reversal on the ECG.*

13. Enter specific information as required by facility into ECG cart.

   a. Correct paper speed is typically 25 mm/second. However, increasing the paper speed will provide a clearer depiction of the waveform morphology. Pediatric cardiologists generally prefer to run the paper at double the speed, 50 mm/second.

14. Press "record" on the ECG cart.

15. Try to eliminate artifact. Repeat ECG if necessary.

16. Remove lead wires from electrodes and electrodes from patient.

17. Discard electrodes and any contaminated material appropriately.

18. Wash your hands.

19. Thank the patient.

20. Document any special information on ECG.

21. Recognize lethal arrhythmia.

22. Maintain confidentiality in all situations.

Quality Assurance/Sources of Error/Limitations

1. Verify Social Security number of patient or assigned institutional number. Use correct Social Security number; some facilities use the Social Security number for serial ECG examinations. Do not transpose digits of number.

     Rationale: *Some patients have inadvertently given their spouses' Social Security numbers.*

2. Recognize and remove artifact.

3. Use fresh electrodes.

     Rationale: *Outdated electrodes will not adhere to skin. Gel will dry out.*

4. Prioritize your time.

5. Document any variation from normal or any information useful to the interpreting physician.

continues

PROCEDURE 1 *continued*

Reporting and Interpreting Results/Documentation

1. Recognize lethal arrhythmias.

2. Report lethal arrhythmia immediately to a nurse or physician for diagnosis and treatment.

3. Document on ECG any physical or extrinsic situation that could alter ECG vector or standard lead placement.

Patient Education

1. Explain briefly that an ECG shows electrical activity relating to how well the heart is pumping, and that it measures such activity through the skin via electrodes attached to lead wires.

2. Assure the patient that the procedure is simple and pain-free, to reduce patient anxiety.

3. Refer patient to physician for actual ECG diagnosis.

REVIEW QUESTIONS

Multiple Choice Questions

1. The epidermis is:
   a. the inner layer of skin.
   b. the middle skin layer.
   c. the outermost layer of skin.

2. The dermis is:
   a. composed of living cells needed to detect ECG signals.
   b. a more resistant and better conducting layer.
   c. a layer of dead skin cells and very conductive for ECG signals.

3. Artifact is:
   a. not the result of inadequate skin preparation.
   b. the result of patient movement.
   c. a straight baseline, not thick and fuzzy.

True/False Questions

_____ 4. The most crucial aspect of ECG performance is patient identification.

_____ 5. It is appropriate for a patient to remain on his side for an ECG if he is asleep.

_____ 6. Excess oil on the skin is removed by using ultrafine sandpaper.

_____ 7. In dextrocardia, the heart is in a mid position in the chest.

_____ 8. Right and left lead reversal should be suspected when the ECG complex is negative in lead I.

_____ 9. Electrodes placed lower than normal need documentation on the ECG.

_____ 10. Tegaderm will assume conductivity if it is applied to open wounds or burns.

_____ 11. It is not necessary to plug the ECG cart into an electrical source when not in use, because the cart has a battery pack.

_____ 12. In dextrocardia, only V1 and V2 electrodes are reversed.

_____ 13. Mentioning the patient's name in conversation harms respect and consideration.

_____ 14. Shaving all chest hair will provide a skin interface for electrode adherence.

_____ 15. Pressure is applied to the center of the electrode for adhesion.

_____ 16. A diagnostic ECG recording requires a current flowing between the epidermis through the conductive gel of the electrode.

_____ 17. Artifact may mimic a number of dysrhythmias, especially atrial and ventricular fibrillation.

_____ 18. Interference in leads II and III may be the result of improper electrode attachment at the left arm site.

_____ 19. If a patient is in a diabetic crisis, it is imperative to perform the ECG at once.

_____ 20. Although used as landmarks for electrode placement, the bones may cause artifact interference.

Learning Activities

21. A patient has just been admitted to the surgical intensive care unit after coronary artery bypass graft surgery. The surgeon has ordered an ECG. What problems will you encounter and how may they be solved?

22. In the emergency department, three patients have been admitted. One is experiencing chest pain and a possible myocardial infarction. The second is in a diabetic coma and the third was in a motor vehicle accident (MVA). The MVA patient is not identified and is unable to speak. Physicians have ordered blood tests and ECGs on all three patients. What will you do and in what order?

23. A patient is in cardiac arrest in the coronary care unit. What will you do to prepare for an ECG order?

24. An emergency department patient is admitted with extreme exposure to cold. She is shaking and trembling. An ECG is ordered by her physician, but the patient refuses. What will you do?